Foreign Medical Graduates

Foreign Medical Graduates

The Case of the United States

Alfonso Mejia
Helena Pizurki
Erica Royston
Division of Health Manpower Development
World Health Organization

Published for
Sandoz Institute for Health and Socio-Economic Studies

by

LexingtonBooks
D.C. Heath and Company
Lexington, Massachusetts
Toronto

This special case study of the United States was sponsored by the World Health Organization. The designations employed and the presentation of material in this publication do not imply the expression of any opinion whatsoever on the part of either the secretariat of the World Health Organization, the Sandoz Foundation, or the Sandoz Institute concerning the legal status of any country, territory, city, or area or of its authorities, or concerning the delimitation of its frontiers or boundaries. The designations used are essentially those indicated in the literature from which the data were retrieved.

Library of Congress Cataloging in Publication Data

Mejia, Alfonso.
Foreign medical graduates.

Part of a multinational study of international migration of physicians and nurses undertaken by the World Health Organization.
Bibliography: p.
1. Physicians, Foreign—United States. 2. Brain drain. I. Pizurki, Helena, joint author. II. Royston, Erica, joint author. III. Sandoz Institute for Health and Socio-Economic Studies. IV. World Health Organization. V. Title. [DNLM: 1. Foreign medical graduates—United States. W76 F715]
R697.F6M43 331.12'7 80-7576
ISBN 0-669-03760-5

Published simultaneously in Canada

Printed in the United States of America

International Standard Book Number: 0-669-03760-5

Library of Congress Catalog Card Number: 80-7576

Jacket by Peter Davies

Contents

List of Figures

List of Tables

Preface

The following observations may be useful to the reader:

1. Much of the physician migration took place at times when certain countries were known by names other than those by which they are known today. In the case of countries where the geographic entity concerned remained the same but only the name of the entity changed, the data on physician migration posed no problem. This would pertain, for example, to Sri Lanka, which was formerly known as Ceylon, and to Democratic Kampuchea, which was formerly known as the Khmer Republic and, before that, as Cambodia.

2. Bangladesh and Pakistan were treated separately when the data allowed. In some cases it was not possible to segregate data referring to what was formerly called Pakistan and had included what is now called Bangladesh. Where this was the case, both entities are designated. Moreover, it is quite possible that a number of migrant physicians who had indicated India as their country of birth and/or medical education were born and/or educated in one or another of the entities that are now respectively designated as Pakistan and Bangladesh.

3. What were formerly designated respectively as the Democratic Republic of Vietnam and the Republic of South Vietnam, but are now unified and called the Socialist Republic of Vietnam, are considered separately because of the considerable difference between the two geographic areas with regard to the rate of physician emigration.

4. China's Province of Taiwan, referred to as Formosa in some reports from which data were retrieved, is treated separately from the mainland of China, that is, the People's Republic of China, because of the considerable difference in the rates of physician migration from the two geographic areas. Even so, the picture may be blurred by the probability that a number of migrant physicians who indicated the Province of Taiwan as their "country of last permanent residence" had indicated "China" as their "country of birth" and/or "country of education." It is worth noting at this point that, in the United States, the country of medical education is what determines whether or not a physician in the United States is a "foreign medical graduate (FMG)," and thus the country of medical education is viewed as the country of origin of the migrant physician, at least insofar as the data of the American Medical Association (AMA) on FMGs are concerned.

5. To the extent possible, the Federal Republic of Germany and the German Democratic Republic were treated separately, as were the Democratic People's Republic of Korea and the Republic of Korea. Where the terms "Germany" or "Korea" were used in the literature to indicate coun-

try of origin, such terms were transferred to those tables in the present document that were based on the literature concerned.

6. Because of the lack of space, and in order to render the text more fluid, the designations of certain countries have been abbreviated. Where this is so, it should be noted that:

D. or Dem. = Democratic

F. or Fed. = Federal

P. = People's

R. or Rep. = Republic

S. or Soc. = Socialist

U. = United

USSR = Union of Soviet Socialist Republics

Abbreviations

AAMC: Association of American Medical Colleges

AHA: American Hospital Association

AMA: American Medical Association

ECFMG: Educational Commission for Foreign Medical Graduates

FLEX: Federation of State Board Licensing Examination

FMG: Foreign Medical Graduate

INS: Immigration and Naturalization Service

USMG: United States and Canadian Medical Graduate

WHO: World Health Organization

Glossary

Accredited Hospital: A U.S. hospital that is certified by the Joint Commission on Accreditation of Hospitals, which is composed of the American Medical Association, the American Hospital Association, the American College of Physicians, and the American College of Surgeons.

Affiliated Hospital: A U.S. hospital that is associated with a medical school which uses that hospital for teaching purposes.

Educational Commission for Foreign Medical Graduates [ECFMG]: A professional organization that combines what was formerly called the Educational Council for Foreign Medical Graduates (established in 1957) and the Commission on Foreign Medical Graduates. Its primary responsibility has been that of evaluating the qualifications of FMGs who desire to enter graduate medical education and health-care programs in the United States. The program of certification administered by the ECFMG includes an examination that tests medical knowledge and English-language proficiency. The examination has been given twice a year in 42 centers in the United States, 7 centers in Canada, and over 125 centers in other countries. ECFMG certification has been applicable to two different but related areas, namely, state licensure and appointment to hospital training programs. With respect to licensure, almost all state licensing boards have listed ECFMG certification as part of the requirements for the permanent licensure of physicians trained outside the United States or Canada, although all but thirteen state boards have allowed waivers in individual cases. With regard to training programs, hospital authorities who wished to maintain approved internship and residency programs and to appoint FMGs to those programs have been required to appoint only those with ECFMG certification or those with a full and unrestricted state license to practice. Similarly, the accreditation of hospitals has been dependent to some extent on the hospital's employing only those FMGs who possessed either valid state licenses or ECFMG certification.

Federation of State Board Licensing Examination [FLEX]: The examination used by all but one or two states to test the eligibility of candidates seeking a license to practice medicine in the state concerned. It is designed for physicians (both FMGs and USMGs) who are in house-staff positions or in practice, and who do not or cannot take the National Board examination.

Foreign Medical Graduate [FMG]: A physician in the United States whose basic medical degree or qualification was conferred by a medical school that is outside the United States, Puerto Rico, and Canada and that is listed in WHO's *World Directory of Medical Schools*. U.S. citizens who obtained their medical education abroad in this sense are considered to be FMGs, while nationals of other countries who graduated from medical schools in the United States, Puerto Rico, and Canada are not.

National Board Examination: A three-part series of examinations offered to students and graduates of approved medical schools of the United States, Puerto Rico, and Canada. Part I examines the candidate's knowledge of six basic medical sciences and is taken after completion of the second year of medical school. Part II examines the candidate's clinical knowledge and is taken after completion of the fourth year of medical school. Part III examines the candidate's clinical judgment and skills and is taken after successful completion of parts I and II and a minimum of six months of internship. While the National Board of Medical Examiners has no authority to issue licenses to practice, most states accept National Board certification, in lieu of their own state board examinations, as a basis for licensure. However, for certification, the National Board has limited its examination to graduates of U.S., Puerto Rican, and Canadian medical schools. Graduates of other medical schools have been required to take the licensure examination given by the state in which they planned practice. (See appendix for recently established regulations regarding the National Board examination as applicable to FMGs.) Both the ECFMG and the FLEX examinations have been constructed largely from testing materials provided by the National Board of Medical Examiners.

United States Medical Graduate [USMG]: A physician in the United States whose basic medical degree or qualification was conferred by a medical school in the United States, Puerto Rico, or Canada. Graduates of Canada's medical schools are considered the same as graduates of U.S. medical schools with respect to professional requirements. Thus, those graduates of Canada's medical schools who are in the United States (6,411 in 1974) are counted as USMGs.

Prologue

For many years concern about the "brain drain" has been reflected in the literature and attested to by numerous resolutions adopted by the United Nations and related specialized agencies—resolutions that have also called for more information on the phenomenon and for measures to modify it in ways desired by governments.

Within the World Health Organization (WHO), concern about the migration of health manpower was expressed at the World Health Assembly and by regional committees; member states requested that WHO undertake a study to identify the patterns of the migration of physicians and nurses and to suggest, with respect to each pattern, alternative measures that could be considered by donor and recipient countries alike.

In response to the World Health Assembly's resolution, WHO undertook a multinational study of the international migration of physicians and nurses, with a view not only to determining the dimensions, directions, and consequences of that migration but also to providing guidance to member states on action they could take to reverse undesirable trends.

This case study of the United States of America, the largest recipient of foreign medical graduates, forms part of that study and offers an insight into the special migration phenomenon that has occurred there over the past decade. It also offers a basis for discussion of possible measures that can be taken by developing countries themselves in order to develop health manpower who will want to stay and work in their own countries.

Health manpower is only one component of health services, into which it must be properly integrated. It is an instrument for effecting health care, but has no meaning in isolation. Health-manpower planning should be based on the country's overall health policies, which in turn should be based on the national political framework; on socioeconomic, educational, and manpower policies; and on an appreciation of national resources and needs.

At present many divergences and discordances exist: between academic and training goals and consumers' expectations and needs; between the goals of training institutions and a country's socioeconomic situation; and between the social goals of health systems and the academic and material expectations of medical graduates and practitioners. In most cases these incongruities result from a lack of communication and collaboration between those responsible for education and training, on the one hand, and health planning and program implementation on the other.

These conditions, existing to some extent in the vast majority of member states, result in the adoption of unsuitable curricula, the use of inappropriate methods and evaluations, and the implementation of irrelevant educational programs. Often the result is the production of disease-oriented professionals instead of health-oriented personnel. In addition, some influential professional groups and leaders have developed hostile attitudes toward any attempt to change the status quo, secondary and tertiary care being more lucrative, prestigious, and glamorous than primary care.

There are many endogenous and exogenous factors that influence the philosophies, curricula, and management systems of training institutions. In addition, there are problems in the field of education itself. Education for any of the health occupations is not, of course, an end in itself; its benefits should be assessed on the basis of its contribution to the improvement of the health status of the population. Education and training for health careers, therefore, must be tailored to match the needs of each country and the health demands of its people. It follows that the needs of the consumers of health services should have a greater influence both on health-training institutions and on the national health administration. These two subsystems—training and administration—must be coordinated and brought into functional integration, with an understanding of the role of each, if they are to respond to the challenge of introducing the necessary changes in both the pattern of health training and the health-care-delivery system.

It is apparent that, while the above concept has been accepted in principle by some international governing bodies, its implementation at the country level has met with considerable resistance and difficulties. A major aim in the area of training, therefore, is to develop feasible methods to permit the introduction of desired changes and the development of training programs along lines that are both appropriate and effective.

Problems can and should be identified, and objectives defined and achieved, only within and by the countries concerned. It is clear that no single activity can solve the problem; a coherent set of actions is needed. Actions will be required in each of the three main areas of the health-manpower process: health-manpower planning; manpower-resources development ("production," education, and training); and health-manpower management. These must be integrated into a single process geared to the development of health services. The realization of this concept of integrated development of health services and health manpower is a precondition of success for any activities undertaken, and will increase the capacity of national health systems to retain practitioners where their services are most needed.

The establishment and functioning of a coordinating device should result in health services that cover the entire population of a country and meet their preventive, curative, and rehabilitative health needs and demands. The services should also be staffed in sufficient numbers by health personnel whose skills have been developed in relation to the country's health problems and possibilities. In this way a comprehensive national health system could be developed that would be fully integrated with all other sectors of community development. Its success, however, will depend on the adequacy of back-up services and of supervisory and referral systems. Appropriate technology is vital for the former; appropriately trained physicians with relevant knowledge, skills, and attitudes are essential members of the latter.

The mutual recognition of health degrees and diplomas, desirable though it may be, obviously facilitates the international migration of professional personnel that has already handicapped so many developing countries. It is for this reason that there would seem to be a basic inconsistency on the part of the World Health Organization, which deplores the migration of physicians but at the same time, knowing the main causal factors of this phenomenon, collaborates with the United Nations Economic and Social Council (UNESCO) to determine criteria for the "equivalence" of medical degrees and diplomas.

For the most part, however, solutions lie in the hands of the developing countries themselves. Only they can develop national strategies and country-specific mechanisms, and forge strong national networks of institutions and programs. Developing countries can also do much to help each other. Through national networks, or components thereof, they can form intercountry relationships and develop technical cooperation; they can also present a united front at international negotiations. Only in this context does the "equivalence" of medical degrees and diplomas have some real value.

As requested by the World Health Assembly, the authors of this book have provided information on the migration phenomenon and have suggested some measures to modify it. Certainly, no new answers will be found by continuing to monitor the flow of health manpower from one country to another. It is now up to member states to act.

D. Tejada-de-Rivero
Assistant Director-General
World Health Organization
Geneva

Introduction

Although foreign medical graduates (FMGs) have for many years been a part of the health-care system in the United States, expressions of concern about their impact in their countries of medical education and the loss they represent to the donor countries began to assume weight only in the early 1970s. That manifestations of concern in the United States were fewer and perhaps less vehement in the 1960s, when the annual inflows first started to increase appreciably, largely reflects the contrast between the country's preoccupation with health-manpower shortages during that period and its current preoccupation with possible surpluses.

Recent health-related legislation in the United States (discussed more fully in the appendix) reflects an attempt to keep the supply of physicians in line with the estimated future demand for medical services. Underlying the legislation is the assumption that, with the accelerated production of domestic graduates in relation to a declining rate of population growth in the United States, a continuing large inflow of FMGs could well convert a potentially adequate supply of physicians into an excess.

As a result of the large annual inflow of physicians since the early 1960s, the proportion of FMGs in the pool of physicians in the United States has increased from 11 percent in 1963 to over 25 percent in 1974. Nearly a third of the filled internship and residency positions throughout the country in 1974 were filled by FMGs, and in recent years almost half of the newly licensed physicians have been products of foreign medical schools. The concern in the United States has centered not only on the sheer numbers of FMGs involved but also on the fact that their presence has not resulted in a more equitable distribution of physicians geographically, institutionally, or in terms of modes of practice and types of services delivered. For the most part, FMGs appear to have followed the pattern of distribution characteristic of graduates of schools in the United States (USMGs) and have thus, if anything, aggravated the problem of maldistribution. Moreover, deep concern has been expressed about the estimated 4,000 to 9,000 FMGs practicing medicine without U.S. licensure.

These facts notwithstanding, there is no denying the invaluable service rendered the American public by FMGs, perhaps not least by those who have been practicing, perhaps without licenses, in areas not particularly appealing to American graduates. What is lamentable is that, for whatever reasons, FMGs have been unable to serve their own countrymen to the same extent.

Most studies of migration have had as one of their objectives the formulation of recommendations as to who should do what about resolving the problem of migration. That was not the intent of this particular case study, one reason being that policy-oriented individuals, groups, and institutions in the United States have been addressing the question of FMGs for a number of years, with the result that the government is now in the process of implementing new legislation aimed at making the country more self-reliant with respect to the supply of health manpower. As for the donor countries, recommendations are implicit in the analyses presented in this case study. Additionally, the report of the WHO multinational study, of which this case study is an extension, contains recommendations relevant to donor countries.

It is worth noting that, even though physician migration to the United States may perforce be reduced considerably as a result of measures now being implemented by the government, the problems will not automatically be resolved with regard to those donor countries that produce more physicians than they can effectively employ. There will always be pull factors somewhere in the world, that is, there will always be countries that both need and can pay for more physicians. To the extent that this is true, there remains the risk that physicians who are either unemployed, underemployed, or inappropriately employed in their homelands will migrate to countries they perceive as offering greater opportunities for professional fulfillment.

Considering the wealth of existing literature on physician migration to the United States, one might question the need for another study. The answer is that, while most studies have viewed the problem only from the standpoint of the United States, this book views it also from the standpoint of the donor countries—in terms both of the factors fostering emigration and of the impact that physician migration to the United States has had on those countries.

This case study is both a part and an extension of the World Health Organization's "Multinational Study of the International Migration of Physicians and Nurses," which was funded by: the Health Resources Administration of the Department of Health, Education, and Welfare (United States); the Educational Commission for Foreign Medical Graduates (United States); the Ministry of Youth, Family Affairs, and Health (Federal Republic of Germany); and the World Health Organization.*

*A. Mejia, H. Pizurki, and E. Royston, *Physician and Nurse Migration: Analysis and Policy Implications* (Geneva: World Health Organization, 1979). Other documents emanating from that study include: "Analytical Review of the Literature" (WHO/HMD/75.7); "Country-Specific Migration Statistics" (WHO/HMD/76.4); "Health Manpower Migration to the Americas" (to be published by the Fogarty International Center as part of its anthology, *Biomedical Research Trends in Latin America and the Caribbean*); and A. Mejia, H. Pizurki, and E. Royston, "Les migrations internationales de médecins et d'infirmières," *Cahiers de Sociologie et de Démographie* 18:101 (1978).

Given this relationship between the present study and the WHO multinational study, the authors of this book would like to acknowledge the contribution to the multinational study made by those members of the WHO staff whose subsequent commitments to other work did not permit a more intimate involvement with this special case study, namely, Barbara Bubb, Barbara Coates, and José Carlos Escudero. Unfortunately, space does not allow us to acknowledge by name the many others who assisted in one way or another with the multinational study, and thus indirectly with the present study. Their assistance is nonetheless fully recognized, and acknowledged with thanks. The study has relied considerably on secondary sources of information; the authors are indebted to those responsible for the individual reports cited as references in this book.

Finally, thanks are due to Dr. Craig D. Burrell, who arranged for financial support for this U.S. case study from the Sandoz Foundation, New York, and to Dr. Philip Selby of the Sandoz Institute, who provided technical assistance in editing and publishing this report.

Although we have endeavored to remain objective in interpreting the data at our disposal, some may disagree with our conclusions. In any case, the conclusions expressed are those of the authors and should in no way be construed as being the responsibility of the organizations that funded either the WHO multinational study or the present study.

Alfonso Mejia
Helena Pizurki
Erica Royston

1 Magnitude and Origins of the Migration

Between one-fifth and one-quarter of all physicians in the United States are foreign medical graduates (FMGs). Almost half of them are from Asian countries, predominantly India and the Philippines. While the number of FMGs more than doubled during the period 1963–1974, in recent years there has been a slowing down in the rate of increase with regard to both the size of the FMG pool and the proportion of the total pool of physicians represented by FMGs.

The United States is an importer not only of medical manpower, that is, physicians born and trained abroad, but also of medical education, that is, physicians who were born in the United States but were trained outside the country; about one-tenth of FMGs are natives of the United States. Asian countries are the largest contributors of medical manpower, while European countries are the largest contributors of medical education.

Among foreign physicians admitted as immigrants to the United States, the number of new arrivals (as opposed to those who changed to immigrant status after spending some time in the United States) was only very slightly greater in the early 1970s than in the late 1960s: about 7,600 per annum in the early 1970s, as opposed to about 7,500 in the late 1960s. Contrary to some assertions, there was no radical decline in the numbers from Europe and no radical increase in the numbers from Asia.

On the basis of data for recent years it has been estimated that, out of every 100 alien FMGs who take the examination of the Educational Commission for Foreign Medical Graduates (ECFMG) for the first time, and thereby perhaps manifest a desire to migrate to the United States, 67 pass the examination; 45 actually arrive in the United States; and 34 achieve licensure to practice in the United States, thereby manifesting an intent to settle in the country.

Not all physicians admitted as immigrants to the United States come directly from their country of birth; for example, of some 7,000 admitted in 1972, about 22 percent were not born in the country they claimed as the place of last permanent residence. Over half of those coming from Canada and over two-thirds of those coming from the United Kingdom were born in an Asian country.

Not all FMGs who come to the United States remain. The departure rate, as estimated by various methods, ranges between 13 and 25 percent per annum. Graduates of Asian schools depart at a higher rate than do those from European and Latin American schools. FMGs who are interns and residents depart at a much higher rate than do FMGs not in training programs.

The outflow of physicians who are citizens of the United States is very small. For every fifty-three foreign-born and foreign-trained physicians in the United States in 1974, one American physician was found abroad.

Pool of FMGs in the United States

Pool in 1974

According to the master file of the American Medical Association (AMA), there were some 83,000 FMGs in the United States in 1974 (table 1-1). Adding the estimated 4,000 to 9,000 FMGs not listed in the master file, one

Table 1-1
Number of Foreign Medical Graduates and Graduates of Canadian Medical Schools in the United States, Specified Years

Year	*Foreign Medical Graduates (1)*	*Graduates of Canadian Medical Schools (2)*	*Total (3)*
1963	30,925	5,644	36,569
1967	45,816	6,050	51,866
1970	57,217	6,174	63,391
1971	62,742	6,446	69,188
1972	68,009	—	—
1973	71,335	6,325	77,660
1974	76,505	6,411	82,916

Sources (for 1963 and 1967): R. Stevens and J. Vermeulen, *Foreign Trained Physicians and American Medicine,* DHEW Publication no. (NIH) 73-325 (Bethesda, Md.: U.S. Department of Health, Education and Welfare, 1972); (1970): American Medical Association, Center for Health Services Research and Development, *Foreign Medical Graduates in the United States,* 1970, ed. J.N. Haug and B.C. Martin (Chicago: American Medical Association, 1971); (1971): K.N. Williams and R.H. Brook, "Foreign Medical Graduates and Their Impact on the Quality of Medical Care in the United States", *Milbank Memorial Fund Quarterly* 53, no. 4(1975):549-579; (1972): American Medical Association, Center for Health Services Research and Development, Profile of Medical Practice; Reference Data, comp. and ed. S.G. Vahovich and P. Aherne (Chicago: American Medical Association, 1973); (1973): American Medical Association, Center for Health Services Research and Development, *Profile of Medical Practice, 75-76,* ed. J. R. Cantwell (Chicago: American Medical Association, 1976); (1974): American Medical Association, 76th Annual Report, "Medical Education in the United States 1975-1976," appendix 1, *Journal of the American Medical Association* 236 (1976):3049-3055.

Note: Figures include U.S.-born FMGs, of whom there were 5,972 (10 percent) in 1970, but exclude FMGs not listed in the AMA's master file (number unknown).

arrives at a total number close to 90,000, or the equivalent of nearly double the number of all physicians, both national and foreign, in Africa in 1974. FMGs constitute over one-fifth of all physicians in the United States.

In 1974 the total number of physicians per 10,000 population in the United States was 17.9, while the number of FMGs per 10,000 population was 3.9. The coverage of population assured in the United States by FMGs alone is greater than that assured by the total number of physicians in most Asian and African countries, including India and the Philippines, the two heaviest contributors of medical manpower to the United States.

In addition to the 76,505 FMGs known to be in the United States in 1974, there were 6,411 graduates of Canadian medical schools. Because the medical education provided in Canada is very similar to that in the United States, those graduates of Canadian schools who are in the United States are not generally included in the statistics on FMGs. A subtraction of their number from the total of FMGs thus leaves some 76,500 who are graduates of schools elsewhere in the world. Of this number about 10 percent are natives of the United States who graduated abroad. The foreign-born FMGs thus numbered some 69,000 in 1974. Because it was not possible to ascertain with any degree of accuracy the number of U.S.-born FMGs, from here onward they are included in the statistics, unless there are indications to the contrary.

Almost half (35,000) of the FMGs in the United States in 1974 came from Asian countries, predominantly the Philippines and India, which together accounted for 19,000 or almost a quarter of the total (tables 1-2 and 1-3).

Table 1-2
Physicians in the United States Who Were Not Graduates of American Medical Schools, by Geographic Area of Graduation, 1970 and 1974

	1970		*1974*	
Geographic Area of Graduation	*Number (1)*	*Percentage (2)*	*Number (3)*	*Percentage (4)*
Africa	1,126	2	1,793	2
Asia	21,002	33	34,930	42
Europe	24,756	39	25,762	31
Canada	6,174	10	6,411	8
Central and South America	9,929	16	13,478	16
Oceania	404	1	542	1
Total	63,391	100	82,916	100

Source: Table 1-3.

Table 1-3
Foreign Medical Graduates in the United States, by Country of Graduation, Specified Years

Country	*1970 (1)*	*1972 (2)*	*1974 (3)*	*Percentage Change 1970–1974 (4)*
Afghanistan	19	24	33	+74
Algeria	1	1	1	0
Argentina	1,313	1,536	1,743	+33
Australia	325	384	430	+32
Austria	1,698	1,670	1,576	−7
Bangladesh	212E[a]	311E	367	+73E
Belgium	511	588	650	+27
Bolivia	146	188	236	+62
Brazil	377	497	619	+64
Bulgaria	49	65	77	+57
Burma	98	155	210	+114
Chile	176	257	363	+106
China (excl. Taiwan)	589	644	655	+11
Colombia	952	1,161	1,251	+31
Costa Rica	11	26	41	+273
Cuba	2,757	2,999	3,200	+16
Czechoslovakia	654	716	720	+10
Dem. Kampuchea			3	
D.P.R. of Korea	5	2	11	+120
D.R. of Vietnam	3	3	3	0
Denmark	82	92	86	+5
Dominican Rep.	629	722	795	+26
Ecuador	147	183	199	+35
Egypt	732	1,006	1,198	+64
El Salvador	91	128	163	+79
Ethiopia	1	1	11	+1,000
Finland	31	42	46	+48
France	685	713	762	+11
German Dem. Rep.	745	700	646	−13
Germany, Fed. Rep. of	3,502	3,508	3,365	−4
Greece	813	919	1,007	+24
Guatemala	109	135	173	+59
Haiti	329	391	439	+33
Honduras	49	65	72	+47
Hong Kong	105	132	144	+37

[a] E = estimate.

Table 1-3 continued

Country	*1970* *(1)*	*1972* *(2)*	*1974* *(3)*	*Percentage Change 1970–1974* *(4)*
Hungary	862	868	852	−1
Iceland	42	49	43	+2
India	3,957	6,303	8,559	+116
Indonesia	89	149	170	+91
Iran	1,631	2,082	2,362	+45
Iraq	188	238	272	+45
Ireland	924	1,024	1,068	+16
Israel	214	281	351	+64
Italy	3,208	3,461	3,584	+12
Jamaica	46	83	122	+165
Japan	882	1,028	903	+2
Lebanon	615	716	757	+23
Malaysia	1	5	7	+600
Malta	6	6	6	0
Mexico	1,821	2,107	2,556	+40
Netherlands	726	746	758	+4
New Zealand	79	100	112	+42
Nicaragua	78	96	109	+40
Nigeria	24	62	91	+279
Norway	44	56	51	+16
Pakistan	572E	841E	1,015	+77E
Panama	23	29	40	+74
Paraguay	76	105	127	+67
Peru	618	754	850	+38
Philippines	7,352	8,846	10,410	+42
Poland	602	747	755	+25
Portugal	107	116	112	+5
Republic of Korea	2,095	2,729	3,479	+66
Republic of Vietnam	12	25	29	+142
Romania	317	395	432	+36
Senegal	1	1	1	0
Singapore	23	40	46	+100
South Africa	356	412	438	+23
Southern Rhodesia	1	1	0	−100
Spain	1,801	2,151	2,357	+31
Sri Lanka	93	263	346	+272
Sudan	2	3	2	0
Surinam	2	2	3	+50
Sweden	54	67	86	+59
Switzerland	2,510	2,564	2,516	0

Table 1-3 continued

Country	*1970* *(1)*	*1972* *(2)*	*1974* *(3)*	*Percentage Change 1970-1974* *(4)*
Syrian Arab Republic	173	270	488	+182
Taiwan	976	1,544	1,888	+93
Thailand	1,098	1,336	1,408	+28
Turkey	866	985	1,014	+17
Uganda	7	31	50	+614
USSR	871	782	850	−2
United Kingdom	2,641	2,764	2,811	+5
Uruguay	46	66	80	+74
Venezuela	133	222	297	+123
Yugoslavia	405	493	546	+35
Zaire	1	1	1	0
Total	57,217	68,009	76,505	+34
Canada	6,174		6,411	+4

Sources (column 1): American Medical Association, Center for Health Services Research and Development, *Foreign Medical Graduates in the United States, 1970*, ed. J.N. Haug and B.C. Martin (Chicago: American Medical Association, 1971), (column 2): idem, *Profile of Medical Practice) Reference Data,* Comp. and ed. S.G. Vahovich and P. Aherne (Chicago: American Medical Association, 1973); (column 3): idem, *Profile of Medical Practice, 75-76*, ed. J.R. Cantwell (Chicago: American Medical Association, 1976).

Notes: Data for Bangladesh and Pakistan were reported separately only for the year 1974, hence estimates were made for each for previous years. See also footnote to table 1-1.

Uncertified FMGs—the "Medical Underground"

As previously indicated, many FMGs are not listed in the AMA's master file. Among them would be some who were neither licensed nor in approved training positions, some who held temporary licenses, and those not in active practice. Estimates of the number involved vary considerably.

Responses to a questionnaire sent to candidates who took the ECFMG examination in the United States in January 1973 showed that 48 percent of the 3,935 candidates who responded were working in the health field at the time of the examination—although such candidates, by definition, were not licensed to practice in the United States. [64] Over half of these respondents indicated that direct patient care was the major component of their work.

From their study of a cohort of FMGs who migrated to the United States during the ten-year period 1961-1971, a research team deduced that about 9,000 or 33 percent of the 27,710 FMGs involved were not listed in the AMA's master file in 1971. [33] This estimate, based on a matching of data from the Immigration and Naturalization Service (INS) with data from the AMA's file, has been strongly challenged by others who, while not criticizing the methodology, did question the interpretation of the data and concluded that a substantial part of the one-third lack of match between the two sets of data was attributable to the departure of a number of FMGs from the United States, to the death of a number, and to technical difficulties in the matching of names. [46]

On the assumption that the AMA's master file accounts for 90 to 95 percent of all FMGs in the United States (a conclusion deriving from the research literature), another research team estimated that there may have been as many as 4,000 to 8,000 FMGs not listed in the AMA's file in 1973. [34]

Changes over Time in the Size of the FMG Pool

The number of FMGs in the United States more than doubled during the period 1963–1974 (table 1–1). Over the last four years of that period, however, the rate of increase was considerably lower than it had been for the first four years, that is, a 34 percent increase for the period 1970–1974 as compared with 48 percent for the period 1963–1967. As shown below, even within the period 1970–1974 the rate of increase had been slowing down:

Years	*Rate of Increase (percent)*
1970–1971	10
1971–1972	8
1972–1973	5
1973–1974	7

A declining rate of increase is also reflected in the proportion of the total physician pool attributable to FMGs (table 1–4). In 1963, FMGs accounted for 11 percent of the pool. Four years later the proportion was 15 percent, an increase of 4 percent. In contrast, the proportion in the 1970s grew more slowly, by about 0.7 percent each year from 1971 onward. Assuming that this rate of growth continued in 1975 and 1976, it can be presumed that in December 1976, that is, just prior to the scheduled implementation date for the new law restricting the inflow of foreign physicians, FMGs numbered about 85,000 (excluding the "underground" and those graduated in Canada) and represented some 22 percent of the total of physicians listed in the AMA's file. There may well have been more, if there is validity in reports that a considerable number of FMGs rushed to the

Table 1-4
Foreign Medical Graduates in the United States: Number, and as a Proportion of the Total Number of Physicians in the United States, Specified Years

Year	Total Number of Physicians (1)[a]	Foreign Medical Graduates: Number (2)[b]	Foreign Medical Graduates: Percentage (3)
1963	275,000	30,900	11
1967	308,000 E[c]	45,800	15
1970	334,000	57,200	17
1971	345,000	62,700	18
1972	357,000	68,000	19
1973	366,000	71,300	19
1974	380,000	76,500	20

Sources (column 1): United States Department of Health, Education, and Welfare, Public Health Service, Health Resources Administration, National Center for Health Statistics, *Health Resources Statistics Reported from the National Center for Health Statistics 1975* (Rockville, Md.: U.S. Department of Health, Education, and Welfare, 1976); (column 2): see table 1-1.

[a]Includes: nonfederal physicians in the fifty states, District of Columbia, Puerto Rico, and other U.S. outlying areas (American Samoa, Canal Zone, Guam, Pacific Islands, and Virgin Islands); those with addresses temporarily unknown to the AMA; and federal physicians in the United States and abroad. Excludes physicians with temporary foreign adresses.

[b]Includes retired physicians and those with addresses temporarily unknown to the AMA; includes U.S.-born FMGs; excludes graduates from Canadian schools.

[c]E = estimate.

United States just prior to 10 January 1977, the date when the restrictions were to come into effect. [9, 26]

Changes over Time in the Composition of the FMG Pool

In addition to changes in the size of the pool of FMGs in the United States, there have also been considerable changes in its composition with respect to region of graduation. (The changes by region are shown in table 1-2, those by country in table 1-3.)

With regard to the distribution of FMGs by region of graduation, the biggest change was in the number from Asia, which increased by nearly 14,000 in four years and, as a proportion of all FMGs, increased from 33 to 42 percent. The next largest increase was in the number from Latin America. All other areas also experienced an increase—Europe very little, Africa and Oceania proportionately more.

Table 1-5
Twelve Countries Contributing the Largest Numbers of Medical Graduates to the United States between 1970 and 1974

Rank[a]	*Country*	*Number Contributed (1)*	*Estimated Number of U.S.-Born Graduates Included (2)*
1	India	4,602	0
2	Philippines	3,058	12
3	Republic of Korea	1,384	0
4	Taiwan	912	2
5	Mexico	735	169
6	Iran	731	0
7	Spain	556	195
8	Egypt	466	1
9	Colombia	447	2
10	Cuba	443	4
11	Pakistan[b]	443 E[c]	0
12	Argentina	430	1

Sources (column 1): table 1-3; (column 2): based on American Medical Association, Center for Health Services Research and Development, *Foreign Medical Graduates in the United States, 1970,* ed. J.N. Haug and B.C. Martin (Chicago: American Medical Association, 1971).

[a] Countries are ranked by size of contribution.

[b] Figures for Pakistan refer to what is now designated as Pakistan.

[c] E = estimate.

That the proportions of the total pool of FMGs deriving from the different regions have changed so much in such a short period of time is quite remarkable, given that the figures involved relate to stock, not inflow. Inasmuch as about three-quarters of the FMGs who have come to the United States have settled there permanently, the existence of such a large core of permanent settlers would normally cause a rather slow rate of change in the composition, by region of origin, of the FMG pool. The drastic changes in the composition observable from table 1-2 reflect the fact that, with respect to region of origin, new entrants to the pool differ considerably from those already in the pool.

Regarding the distribution of FMGs by country of graduation, the biggest increases by far were in the numbers from India, the Philippines, and the Republic of Korea—all Asian countries. In fact, when countries are ranked by the magnitude of increase in absolute numbers (table 1-5), five of the first six countries are Asian—the three mentioned above plus Iran and China's Province of Taiwan. Spain is a special case, in that many FMGs from Spain are not Spanish nationals. For example, of the 1,801 FMGs in the United States in 1970 who were graduates of Spain's medical schools, 622 (over a third) were born in the United States. [3] Almost certainly, many of the remainder were also not nationals of Spain. (The relationships between country of education, country of citizenship, and country of birth of FMGs are elaborated in the next section. The relationship between country of birth and country of last permanent residence is discussed later in this chapter.)

Origins of the Pool of FMGs

For many physicians, migration is not a once-and-for-all move from one country to another. Evidence shows that it is possible for an individual to be born in one country; obtain basic professional education in another country; pursue graduate education in a third country; and either remain in that country, move to yet another country, or return to either the country of birth or the country of education. Such mobility, combined with the fact that the AMA's statistics classify physicians in the United States by country of basic medical education, leads to confusion with regard to the national origins not only of the physicians who graduated abroad—the FMGs—but also of those alien physicians in the United States who had obtained their basic medical education in the United States. The latter, those graduating in the United States, are counted not as FMGs but as USMGs, whose number thus includes both aliens and American citizens. How many USMGs are aliens is not apparent from the statistics, but the number is probably small. While some data are available on the number of foreign medical students in the United States at a given time or another—for example, about 800 in the academic year 1973-1974, according to a study by UNESCO—no data are available on the number of such students who, after graduation, either remain in the United States or, after leaving the United States, return at a later date. [53] In both cases, such graduates would be classified as USMGs, and their identities as nationals of other countries would thus be lost in the statistics.

The confusion regarding the national origins of the FMGs arises from the fact that a graduate of a particular country X may also be one of the following:

1. currently a citizen of country X;
2. originally a citizen of country X but currently a naturalized citizen of the United States;
3. a citizen by birth of the United States;
4. currently a citizen of a third country, country Y; or

5. originally a citizen of country Y but currently a naturalized citizen of the United States.

Part of the confusion, directly related to the above characteristics of the FMG pool, is the difficulty of gauging the extent to which certain countries are exporters of *medical education* as opposed to *medical manpower,* and the extent to which the United States is an importer in each of these respects. The following definitions of exportation and importation with respect to FMGs in the United States may be useful for an understanding of the subsequent analyses:

1. A country is considered as having *exported medical education* to the extent that it provided such education to citizens of another country who thereafter joined the pool of FMGs in the United States.
2. A country is considered as having *exported medical manpower* to the extent that those of its citizens who obtained their medical education within the country thereafter joined the pool of FMGs in the United States.
3. The United States is considered as having *imported medical education* to the extent that those of its citizens who obtained their medical education abroad thereafter returned and joined the pool of FMGs in the United States.
4. The United States is considered as having *imported medical manpower* to the extent that its pool of FMGs contains physicians who had not obtained their medical education in the United States and were not natives of the United States.

The most recent report available that provides notions of the relationship between country of medical education and country of citizenship is that of a study of a cohort of FMGs who were listed in the AMA's file in 1968 but not in 1966. [13] Table 1-6, which comes from that report, shows two contrasting phenomena: (1) when the cohort was viewed from the standpoint of region of citizenship, it was found that, of those FMGs who were citizens of a country in Europe, Asia, or Latin America, about 90 percent had also obtained their medical education in their country of citizenship; and (2) when the cohort was viewed from the standpoint of region of medical education, it was found that, of those who obtained their medical education in a country of Europe, Asia, or Latin America, only 64 percent were citizens of their country of medical education. The difference arises partly because FMGs, when classified by country of medical education, include those who are citizens of countries other than the country of medical education, among them native and naturalized citizens of the United States.

When FMGs are classified by region of citizenship, Latin America's

Table 1–6
Relationship between Citizenship Status and Country of Medical Education of Foreign Medical Graduates Who Entered the United States between Year End 1966 and 1968

	A. Region of Citizenship (percent)			
	Europe *N = 1,239*	*Asia* *N = 4,387*	*Latin America* *N = 1,902*	*Canada* *N = 268*
Educated in country of citizenship	88	92	89	88
Educated in region of citizenship	93	98	93	88
Educated in region but not country of citizenship	5	7	5	—
Educated outside region of citizenship	7	2	7	12
	B. Region of Medical Education			
	Europe *N = 3,167*	*Asia* *N = 4,984*	*Latin America* *N = 2,401*	*Canada* *N = 1,025*
Citizen of country of medical education	1,088 (34%)	4,019 (81%)	1,686 (70%)	235 (23%)
Citizen of region of medical education	1,152 (36%)	4,313 (87%)	1,776 (74%)	235 (23%)
Citizenship other than country of medical education:				
Europe	64	47	16	3
Asia	57	294	8	2
Latin America	117	7	89	1
Canada	30	3	0	—
Native United States	495	14	70	180
Naturalized United States	744	81	149	207
Other	88	7	10	1
Missing data	484	512	373	396

Source: I. Butter, "The Migratory Flow of Doctors to and from the United States," *Medical Care* 9(1971):17–31.

contribution of native manpower (including both those trained in Latin America and those trained elsewhere) is shown to be substantially larger in absolute numbers than that of Europe, a fact not evident when the classification is by country of medical education, as is the case with AMA data. On the other hand, Europe is for the most part an exporter of medical education, as is Canada, although smaller numbers are involved in the latter case. In both cases, however, the exported education was primarily that given to native and naturalized citizens of the United States. The latter category may well include those who were formerly citizens of the country of graduation. Asia contributes the largest absolute amount of domestically trained medical manpower; 87 percent of the FMGs trained in Asian countries were also citizens of Asian countries.

Table 1-7, which is derived from data in the previously mentioned report, shows some interesting differences between individual countries with regard to the citizenship status and the country of education of FMGs. By adding, for each country, the figure in column 3 to that in column 4, one can readily see that the countries that are predominantly exporters of medical education as opposed to medical manpower are, in proportional terms and descending order of magnitude, Spain (60 percent), Formosa (58 percent), Switzerland (52 percent), Italy (49 percent), France (47 percent), Belgium (43 percent), and Ireland (39 percent). Of these, Belgium, Italy, Spain, and Switzerland exported primarily the education they provided for American citizens. France and Formosa, on the other hand, exported primarily the education they provided for citizens of other countries. In this respect, table 1-7 highlights a feature that is not apparent in other data sets, namely, the extent to which certain countries are providers of medical education to those citizens of other countries who subsequently migrate to the United States.

The figures in column 2 of table 1-7 show, again for 1968, the proportion of those FMGs concerned who were naturalized citizens of the United States. On the assumption that these were originally natives of the country of medical education (although this may not be so in all cases), one can combine the first two columns, the sum of which gives an indication of the extent to which the country concerned is exporting medical manpower as distinct from medical education. Thus, with the exception of Formosa, most Asian countries are *not* exporters of medical education, while most countries of Europe are.

It is also interesting to note from table 1-7 the high percentages of naturalized citizens of the United States among those FMGs who graduated from schools in Austria, Czechoslovakia, Germany, Hungary, China, and the Dominican Republic. While the country of birth of these graduates is not indicated, it is likely that most of them are old graduates of those countries who were also born in their country of graduation. The author of the report cites China and Formosa (that is, China's Province of Taiwan) as being somewhat atypical, in that the FMGs from Formosa include more Chinese than Formosan citizens as well as six times as many Chinese citizens as there are among the FMGs who graduated in China; of those who graduated in Formosa, only 34 percent are Formosan citizens as opposed to 52 percent who are citizens of the mainland of China.

Table 1-7
Relationship between Country of Medical Education and Citizenship Status of Foreign Medical Graduates Who Entered the United States between Year End 1966 and 1968, Selected Countries

	Percentage of FMGs Trained in the Country Who Are:				
Region and/or Country of Medical Education	*Also Its Citizens (1)*	*Naturalized Citizens of United States (2)*	*Citizens by Birth of United States (3)*	*Citizens of Other Countries (4)*	*Unidentified by Citizenship (5)*
Europe					
Austria	12	55	1	11	12
Belgium	33	9	40	3	14
Czechoslovakia	41	34	2	6	16
France	14	15	15	32	24
Germany	28	48	6	6	12
Greece	50	18	5	6	21
Hungary	14	55	—	14	17
Ireland	32	5	12	27	24
Italy	14	23	42	7	14
Poland	52	24	2	9	13
Spain	23	9	35	25	8
Switzerland	23	16	38	14	9
Turkey	68	3	0	4	24
United Kingdom	59	9	6	6	20
Australia	65	6	1	8	20
Canada	23	20	18	1	38
Asia					
China	41	22	1	27	9
Formosa	34	1	—	58	7
India	90	0	—	3	6
Iran	85	1	—	1	
Japan	76	1	1	5	17
Korea	90	2	0	1	7
Pakistan	84	—	—	8	8
Philippines	80	2	0	3	14
Thailand	93	0	—	1	6
Middle East					
Egypt	65	1	—	20	14
Israel	85	2	—	4	10

Table 1-7 continued

Region and/or Country of Medical Education	Percentage of FMGs Trained in the Country Who Are: Also Its Citizens (1)	Naturalized Citizens of United States (2)	Citizens by Birth of United States (3)	Citizens of Other Countries (4)	Unidentified by Citizenship (5)
Latin America					
Argentina	75	3	0	9	13
Brazil	86	2	—	2	10
Colombia	66	1	—	2	31
Cuba	75	12	1	0	12
Dominican Republic	60	22	3	2	13
Mexico	53	6	16	12	13
Peru	84	1	1	11	13
Other		11	1	74	14
Total	55	10	6	13	16

Source: Derived from data in I. Butter, "The Migratory Flow of Doctors to and from the United States," *Medical Care* (1971):17-31.

Notes: Names of countries are as given in the source. A zero represents less than 0.5 percent. A dash means none. Percentages do not add to 100 because of rounding. In columns 1-3 percentages include FMGs whose citizenship was ascertainable and thus may be underestimates. Naturalized U.S. citizens who graduated in a specified country may or may not have originally been citizens of that country.

While table 1-7 shows that only about 6 percent of the FMGs in the study were citizens by birth of the United States and thus recipients of imported education, data for 1970 show that about 10 percent of all FMGs in the United States are recipients of imported education. Table 1-8, which is based on AMA data, indicates the extent to which the United States imports medical education from individual countries. [3] By far the largest number of U.S.-born FMGs were trained in Italy and Switzerland (some 1,300 in each), followed by the United Kingdom and Spain with half that number each, and then by Mexico with slightly fewer. These are essentially the countries from which the *United States* imports medical education; but not all of them are predominantly exporters of medical education in general. Of those mentioned above, neither Mexico nor the United Kingdom ranks high among the exporters listed in table 1-7.

A comparison of table 1-7 (column 3) with table 1-8 shows a considerable difference in the proportions of natives of the United States among the FMGs trained in Switzerland, the United Kingdom, Mexico, and Austria. For all four countries, the proportion of U.S. natives in the total pool of FMGs in 1970 (table 1-8) was considerably higher than that in the cohort joining the pool between 1966 and 1968 (table 1-7). It would be interesting

Table 1-8
Major Exporters of Medical Education to the United States, 1970

	Foreign Medical Graduates		
Country of Graduation	*Total Number (1)*	*Number Born in United States (2)*	*Percentage Born in United States (2) ÷ (1) (3)*
Italy	3,208	1,375	43
Switzerland	2,510	1,338	53
United Kingdom	2,641	667	25
Spain	1,801	622	35
Mexico	1,821	413	23
Germany, Federal Republic of	3,502	253	7
Netherlands	726	232	32
Belgium	511	208	41
Austria	1,698	194	11
Ireland	924	151	16
France	685	115	17
German Democratic Republic	745	53	7
Greece	813	41	5
Other countries	35,632	310	1
Total	57,217	5,972	10

Source: American Medical Association, Center for Health Research and Development, *Foreign Medical Graduates in the United States, 1970,* ed. J.N. Haug and B.C. Martin (Chicago: American Medical Association, 1971).

Notes: Figures exclude graduates of medical schools in Canada, which totalled 6,174 in 1970 and of which the number and percentage born in the United States were not indicated in the above source.

to know whether these differences reflect the possibility that more U.S. natives who were trained in these countries joined the pool *after* rather than *before* the 1966-1968 cohort, or vice versa.

While figures such as those in the above-mentioned tables show the proportions of FMGs who are not natives of the country of graduation, they do not tell much about the actual country of birth of such FMGs, excepting those born in the United States. The AMA's early census of physicians in the United States would no doubt yield such information. The cohort study mentioned above used that census, but only for a limited population of FMGs—the 12,072 FMGs who joined the pool between the end of 1966 and the end of 1968. [13] In that study it was found, for example, that among the 367 graduates from Spain, there were 62 Cubans, 7 Dominican Republicans, 5 Peruvians, 3 Colombians, 1 Belgian, 1 Greek, 1 Indian, 130 U.S. natives, 32 naturalized Americans, and only 84 Spaniards (not

Table 1–9
Standard ECFMG Certificate: Number Issued in United States in 1974 and Distribution of Recipients by Country of Medical School and by Country of Citizenship at Time of Entrance to Medical School

	Country of:			
	Medical School		*Citizenship*	
	Number	*Percentage*	*Number*	*Percentage*
United States			166	2
Argentina	120	2	116	1
Australia	147	2	126	2
Brazil	101	1	95	1
China-Taiwan	249	3	197	3
Cuba	74	1	100	1
Germany, Fed. Rep. of	161	2	143	2
India	1,753	23	1,697	22
Iran	198	3	207	3
Italy	91	1	45	1
Japan	224	3	214	3
Korea	420	5	417	5
Mexico	182	2	134	2
Pakistan	189	2	207	3
Philippines	900	12	855	11
Spain	109	1	73	1
Switzerland	106	1	73	1
Thailand	141	2	148	2
United Arab Republic	133	2	83	1
United Kingdom	190	2	256	3
Other	2,256	30	2,459	32
Total	7,579	100	7,579	100

Source: Educational Commission for Foreign Medical Graduates, *Annual Report, 1974* (Philadelphia: Educational Commission for Foreign Medical Graduates 1976).
Note: Designations of countries are as indicated in the source.

counting those there might be among the naturalized Americans); there were also 41 whose nationality was not specified.

Some measure of the citizenship status of new entrants or would-be entrants to the FMG pool can be obtained from an analysis of the distribution of recipients of the Standard ECFMG Certificate. Table 1–9 shows the distribution, by country of medical education and by country of citizenship, of those receiving the certificate in 1974. In most cases, more of the recipients were graduates of the specified country than were citizens thereof. This is attributable to the fact that nearly 500 (or 7 percent) of the recipients had obtained medical education outside their country of citizenship, among them 166 Americans and 203 from unspecified countries. Some of the latter may have studied abroad because there was no medical school in their homeland.

While it is not surprising that Italy, Mexico, Spain, and Switzerland are among the group that had more graduates than citizens in the population receiving certificates in the United States (given that they have traditionally been heavy exporters of medical education), it is interesting to note that, among the graduates from China (Taiwan) and Egypt, a relatively high proportion represents the exportation of medical education: 21 and 38 percent, respectively. Among the countries listed, those with more citizens than graduates were Cuba, Iran, Pakistan, Thailand, and the United Kingdom.

Unfortunately, the percentage distribution in table 1-9 cannot be used to estimate the distribution of the current pool of FMGs, because it is unlikely that new entrants or would-be entrants to the pool would have the same characteristics as FMGs who have been in the United States for many years.

Inflow of FMGs

While a comparison of data on the pool of FMGs at various points in time provides a fairly clear picture of the growth of the pool, it does little to explain the dynamic nature of the pool, that is, the proportion that constitutes a hard core of permanent migrants and the proportion that comes and goes, causing a constantly changing pool. Published data reveal very little information on the subject. AMA data reflect merely a head count, with no indication as to what proportion of the heads is the same at each count.

Some notion of the mobility of FMGs can be gleaned from other types of data, such as data collected by the Immigration and Naturalization Service (INS), which show the numbers of foreign physicians entering the United States, but not the numbers leaving; data on the numbers of FMGs being licensed, which probably give a fair indication of the numbers intending to settle in the United States; data on the numbers of FMGs sitting for the ECFMG examination, which probably give a fair notion of the numbers desiring entry into the United States; and data deriving from studies of various cohorts of FMGs. In the following analyses, such pieces of information will be used to provide some notion of the mobility of FMGs.

Numbers Entering the United States

In order to understand the sharp increases observed in the past few years with regards to the inflow of foreign physicians to the United States, it is essential to understand the ways in which the statistics on inflow are calculated. To this end, it is essential to understand the various avenues of entry that have been available to foreign physicians. While these are discussed in greater detail in the appendix, for the purpose of the analysis that follows, it may suffice to know that one avenue is the "immigrant" route, whereby the physician is admitted as a permanent resident at the moment of initial entry to the United States, either for employment or for educational purposes. The second is the "nonimmigrant" route, whereby the physician enters with a temporary visa, with the option of having it converted to a permanent or immigrant visa at a later date. Statistics on the annual inflow of foreign physicians to the United States are blurred by the fact that the number recorded as entering as *immigrants* during a given year include both the number of new entrants and the number of those physicians who had previously entered with temporary (nonimmigrant) visas but had these converted to permanent (immigrant) visas during the given year. These statistics give the impression that the annual number of new entrants has been rising at a rapid pace.

Table 1-10, which provides basic data on the annual inflow of foreign physicians during the period 1965-1973, shows that the number of those recorded as being admitted as immigrants includes a substantial number of physicians who, having initially entered as nonimmigrants, later converted to immigrant status. With regard to the numbers and proportions who did this, two distinct periods can be identified. The first is the period beginning in 1966, that is, the year following the passage of the Immigration Act of 1965, which replaced the system of unequal national quotas with a more flexible one that placed a premium on skills rather than on national origins. The second is the period beginning in 1971, the year following the passage of a law that virtually abolished the requirement that exchange visitors who wanted to become immigrants first had to leave the United States for two years. During both periods, there were sharp increases in both the number and the proportion of immigrant physicians who were not new arrivals but who had adjusted their visa status. The number of immigrants who were new arrivals also increased, but at a much slower rate. Moreover, their number as a proportion of the total declined from 94 percent to 42 percent in 1973, which means that the overcount was growing proportionately each year. To the extent that all foreign physicians admitted as immigrants were presumed to be new arrivals, the data in table 1-10 show that, for the period 1965-1973, there was an overcount of nearly 15,000, representing the number who changed status.

In addition to the new arrivals among the immigrant group, there was a considerable but fairly even flow of other new arrivals—those arriving as nonimmigrants, primarily as exchange visitors. When their total is added to the total of newly arriving immigrants, it can be seen that the increases in the annual inflow of new arrivals, particularly for the years beginning in

Table 1-10
Relationship between the Number of Foreign Physicians Newly Entering the United States and the Number Whose Visa Status Was Adjusted; and Relationship between the Number of Newly Entering Foreign Physicians and the Number of Students Graduating from Medical Schools in the United States, 1965–1973

	Immigrants						
Fiscal Year	*Number Recorded (1)*	*Number Adjusting Visa (2)*	*Number New Entrants (1) − (2) (3)*	*Total Number Nonimmigrants (4)*	*Total New Entrants (3) + (4) (5)*	*Previous Estimates (6)*	*Total Medical Students Graduating in United States (7)*
1965	2,012	112	1,900	4,114	6,014	6,382	7,409
1966	1,549	474	2,075	4,553	6,628	7,105	7,574
1967	3,325	841	2,484	5,631	8,115	8,897	7,743
1968	3,060	652	2,408	5,997	8,405	9,125	7,973
1969	2,756	576	2,180	4,759	6,939	7,515	8,059
1970	3,155	890	2,265	5,365	7,630	8,523	8,367
1971	5,748	2,902	2,846	5,033	7,879	10,789	8,974
1972	7,143	4,389	2,754	4,270	7,024	11,417	9,551
1973	7,119	4,140	2,979	5,144	8,123	12,262	10,391
Total	36,867	14,976	21,891	44,866	66,757	82,015	76,041

Source: R. Stevens et al., "Physician Migration Reexamined," *Science* 190(1975):439–442.

1971, were much smaller than those inferred from previous estimates (column 5 compared with column 6 in table 1-10). Additionally, and contrary to the notion that the annual inflow of new arrivals exceeded the annual production of physicians in the United States, the data show that this was so only for the years 1967 and 1968. For all other years, the opposite was the case: the number of physicians produced locally was greater than the number of new arrivals.

The factor of visa-status adjustments is particularly important in checking assertions that the pattern of inflow has been changing radically with respect to regions of origin. From table 1-11, which is derived from the same source as table 1-10, [48] it can be seen that, assertions to the contrary, there was no radical decline in the numbers of new arrivals from Europe and no radical increase in the numbers from Asia. However, the numbers from Latin America increased both absolutely and proportionally. There was also a steady rise in the flow from Africa, although both numerically and proportionally the numbers were low. With regard to the total number of new arrivals, the number arriving during the period 1970–1973 was only slightly greater than that in the four preceding years—30,656 or about 7,600 per annum, versus 30,087 or 7,500 per annum.

As far as Asia is concerned, the notion that the number of new arrivals was rapidly increasing arose from the fact, unknown to most observers, that among the physicians recorded as immigrants were many who had already been residing in the United States but were merely changing their visa status. As an illustration of this phenomenon, table 1-12 shows for a single year (1972) the number and proportion of immigrant physicians from each region who were direct immigrants, as opposed to those who converted from nonimmigrant status. With regard to Asia, for every direct immigrant there were more than two who represented a change in status. In fact, of all the immigrants representing a change in status, the vast majority were from Asia (3,861, or 88 percent, of a total of 4,389).

Numbers Intending to Enter the United States

While data on the numbers of a country's physicians who are actually living abroad at particular points in time are the best available indicator of the volume of emigration from that country, it is important to have some notion of the number that might have been interested in going abroad if the opportunity to do so had materialized. One indication of such possible interest, as it pertains to migration to the United States, is the number of foreign medical graduates who took the ECFMG examination during the years when passing that examination amounted to eligibility for appointment to an accredited graduate medical-education program in the United

Table 1-11
New Entries of Immigrant and Nonimmigrant Physicians into the United States, by Continents, 1965-1973[a]

	North and Central America		*South America*		*Europe*		*Asia*		*Africa*		*All Other Areas*		*Total*	
Fiscal Year	*Number*	*Percent-age*	*Number*	*Percent-age*	*Number*	*Percent-age*	*Number*	*Percent-age*	*Number*	*Percent-age*	*Number*	*Percent-age*	*Number*	*Percent-age*
1965	1,282	21	528	9	1,567	26	2,376	40			261	4	6,014	100
1966	1,206	18	538	8	1,637	25	2,980	45			267	4	6,628	100
1967	1,147	14	562	7	2,211	27	3,838	47	207	3	150	2	8,115	100
1968	1,228	15	706	8	2,002	24	4,157	49	219	3	93	1	8,405	100
1969	959	14	526	7	1,722	25	3,331	48	273	4	128	2	6,939	100
1970	1,031	13	599	8	1,922	25	3,571	47	365	5	142	2	7,630	100
1971	1,221	16	821	10	1,359	17	4,106	52	303	4	69	1	7,879	100
1972	920	13	737	10	1,367	20	3,630	52	274	4	96	1	7,024	100
1973	1,193	15	946	11	1,598	20	3,754	46	471	6	161	2	8,123	100
Total	10,187	15	5,963	9	15,385	23	31,743	48	2,112	3	1,367	2	66,757	100

Source: R. Stevens et al., "Physician Migration Reexamined," *Science* 190(1975):439-442.

Note: African entrants for 1965 and 1966 are included under "All other areas."

[a] Immigrants are counted according to country of birth, nonimmigrants according to country of last permanent residence.

Table 1-12
Foreign Physicians Admitted as Immigrants to the United States, by Region of Birth and Visa Status, 1972

		Foreign Physicians			
		Adjusted Visas		*New Entrants*	
Region of Birth	*Total Admitted (1)*	*Number (2)*	*Percentage (3)*	*Number (4)*	*Percentage (5)*
Europe	654	326	50	328	50
Americas	626	47	8	579	92
Asia	5,558	3,861	69	1,697	31
Africa	259	128	49	131	51
Oceania	46	27	59	19	41
Total	7,143	4,389	61	2,754	39

Source: K.N. Williams and B.A. Lockett, "Migration of Foreign Physicians to the United States: The Perspective of Health Manpower Planning," *International Journal of Health Services* 4(1974):213-243.

States. In fact, with only rare exceptions, foreign medical graduates could not *legally* practice medicine in the United States unless they had passed that examination.

Table 1-13 shows the numbers of those taking and those passing the ECFMG examination during the period 1958-1974. A comparison of column 1 of that table with column 5 of table 1-10 shows that, in contrast to the numbers of new arrivals to the United States, the numbers each year taking the examination for the first time had grown considerably—increasing from about 9,800 per annum during the period 1960-1964 to about 17,400 per annum during the period 1970-1974, a rise of nearly 78 percent. Regarding the number passing the examination, which is a more accurate indicator of the potential flow to the United States, the average number per annum increased from 6,000 during the period 1960-1964 to 12,300 in 1970-1974, or double that of the earlier period.

A comparison of the numbers passing the ECFMG examination with the numbers of new arrivals to the United States (table 1-10) shows, however, that the former is a very poor predictor of the latter. While there is some correlation between the two with regard to fluctuations (with a one-year time lag), there is very little relationship regarding the trend (see figure 1-1). A much more interesting correlation emerging from figure 1-1 is that between the numbers achieving immigrant status (table 1-10, column 1) and the numbers becoming licensed in the United States (again, with a time lag of about a year). This relationship would seem to indicate that, although the

Table 1-13
Examinations Given by the Educational Council for Foreign Medical Graduates, 1958-1974

Year	*First Examination (1)*	*Repeat Examination (2)*	*Total Examinations (3)*	*Number Passing (4)*	*Percentage Passing (5)*
1958	1,094	48	1,142	570	50
1959	4,477	363	4,840	2,139	44
1960	11,301	3,467	14,768	5,773	39
1961	8,204	6,018	14,222	5,381	38
1962	8,906	5,629	14,535	6,054	42
1963	11,391	7,739	19,130	6,043	32
1964	9,378	9,133	18,511	6,280	37
1965	9,204	9,133	18,337	7,724	42
1966	10,765	8,223	18,988	7,842	41
1967	11,777	7,411	19,188	8,820	46
1968	11,975	7,753	19,548	7,774	40
1969	12,447	10,151	22,598	8,127	36
1970	16,631	13,319	29,950	11,916	40
1971	16,525	14,508	31,033	9,693	31
1972	15,556	16,516	32,072	12,837	40
1973	18,694	18,329	37,023	12,289	33
1974	19,711	17,736	37,447	14,868	39

Sources (1958-1973): United States Bureau of Health Resources Development, Office of International Health Manpower Studies, *Foreign Medical Graduates and Physician Manpower in the United States*, DHEW Publication no, (HRA) 74-30 (Bethesda, Md.: U.S. Department of Health, Education, and Welfare, 1974; (1974): Educational Commission for Foreign Medical Graduates, *Financial Report, 1974* (Philadelphia: Educational Commission for Foreign Medical Graduates, 1976).

numbers of foreign physicians achieving immigrant status is a poor predictor of new additions to the FMG pool, it is a good predictor of the numbers intending to settle in the United States, which is the subject of the next section of this report.

Numbers Intending to Settle in the United States

Perhaps one of the strongest indicators of the intention of foreign physicians to settle in the United States can be found in the numbers seeking a license to practice medicine in the United States. Those seeking the license are required, among other things, to pass a licensing examination. Table

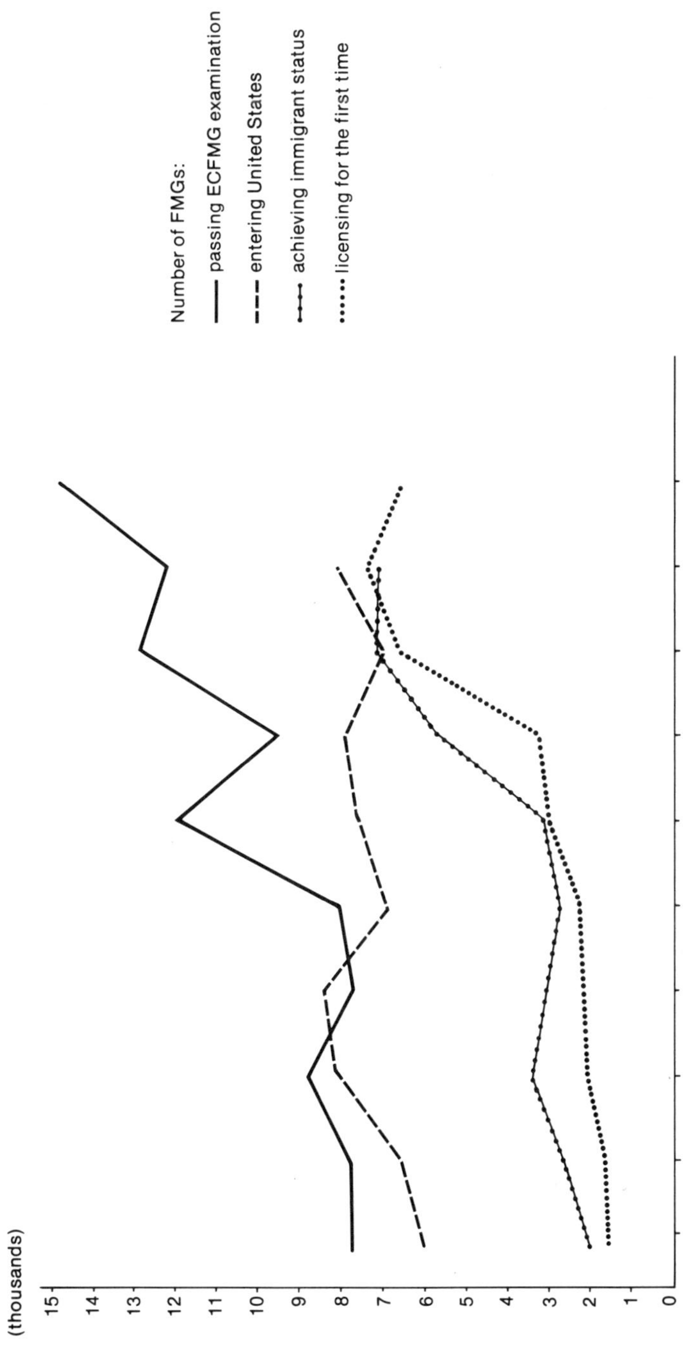

Figure 1–1. Trends in Physician Migration.

1-14 shows that the number taking that examination in 1971 and in 1972 was about four times the number in 1955, and about three times that in 1965.

As an illustration of the countries of origin (in this case, countries of graduation) of the candidates for licensure, figures for the year 1972 are presented below. [54] The figures can be taken only as a rough guide for reasons noted in the footnote to table 1-14.

Region of Graduation	*Numbers of FMGs Examined*
Europe	1,394
Central and South America	1,474
Asia	5,955
Africa	250
Oceania	42
Total	9,115

The 9,115 FMGs taking the examination in 1972 comprised graduates from eighty countries. Those countries having the most (75 or more) candidates that year were, according to regions:

Europe	
Spain	212
Italy	168
Turkey	127
Germany	105
United Kingdom	89
Greece	88
Poland	81
Yugoslavia	75
Americas	
Cuba	472
Colombia	223
Mexico	193
Argentina	165
Peru	85

Africa	
Egypt	207
Asia	
Philippines	2,149
India	1,226
Korea	716
Taiwan	427
Iran	424
Thailand	295
Pakistan	238

Of candidates from the countries cited, those from Spain, Italy, and Mexico most probably included a large proportion of FMGs born in the United States.

As can be seen from table 1-14, however, not all those who took the examination passed. The failure rate averaged nearly 50 percent in the years prior to 1960 and about 35 percent thereafter. What happens to those who fail is not documented—some may leave the United States and, of those

Table 1-14
U.S. Licensure Examinations Administered to Foreign Medical Graduates, Specified Years between 1935 and 1972

Year	Number Examined (1)	Number Passing (2)	Percentage Failing (3)
1935	437	303	31
1940	2,088	948	55
1945	475	209	56
1950	799	359	55
1955	1,771	1,042	41
1960	2,864	2,013	30
1965	3,011	2,043	32
1966	3,691	2,281	38
1967	4,187	2,590	38
1968	4,936	3,100	37
1969	4,911	3,164	36
1970	6,236	3,911	37
1971	10,380	6,747	35
1972	9,115	5,817	36

Sources (1935–1970): R. Stevens and J. Vermeulen, *Foreign Trained Physicians and American Medicine*, DHEW Publication no. (NIH) 73-325 (Bethesda, Md.: U.S. Department of Health, Education, and Welfare, 1972); (1971–1972): United States, Bureau of Health Resources Development, Office of International Health Manpower Studies, *Foreign Medical Graduates and Physician Manpower in the United States*, DHEW Publication no. (HRA) 74-30 (Bethesda, Md.: U.S. Department of Health, Education, and Welfare, 1974).

Notes: Figures include U.S.-born FMGs. Graduates from Canadian schools are excluded. The figures should be viewed only as a rough guide, given that candidates who fail tend to retake the examination at a later date, and some candidates take the examination in more than one state, often in the same year. The result is that the total number of graduates involved is overestimated.

who remain, some may continue to study; others may seek work in the health field that requires no license; and others may work outside the health field. A substantial number retake the examination.

Passing the licensure examination is only one of the requirements to be met by alien FMGs seeking permission to practice legally in the United States. Others include ECFMG certification and either American citizenship or, in lieu of that, an immigrant visa or a declaration of intent to become a citizen. The requirements vary from state to state. Table 3-13 shows the numbers of alien FMGs who apparently met the various requirements and were thus added to the pool of medical licentiates in the United States. From that table it can also be seen that, during recent years, some 6,000 alien FMGs annually had become medical licentiates, thereby manifesting an intent to settle permanently in the United States. This number is closely related to the number of FMGs achieving immigrant status, another indicator of intent to settle (see figure 1-1).

On the basis of annual averages for the years 1970-1974, a comparison of the number of new licentiates (6,000) with the number of FMGs taking the ECFMG examination for the first time (17,400), the number passing that examination (11,700), and the number of new arrivals to the United States (7,600), suggests that, for every 100 FMGs taking the ECFMG examination for the first time, 67 pass the test, 45 arrive in the United States, and 34 achieve licensure and thereby manifest an intent to settle.

Way Stations

Not all physicians admitted as immigrants to the United States come directly from their country of birth. Many enter via another country, either because they had received their medical qualifications in a country other than their country of birth (see the section on the origins of the pool of FMGs) or other reasons—political, economic, professional, and so on. For the individuals who display such migration behavior, certain countries can be said to function as way stations. The countries that physicians use as way stations can to some extent be distinguished from the countries of origin of such physicians from data on physicians admitted to the United States as immigrants in 1972.

From table 1-15 it can be seen that the main way stations, in terms of absolute numbers of foreign physicians passing through these countries to the United States, were Canada, the United Kingdom, and China's Province of Taiwan. It is also interesting to note that, in the case of two countries, Saudi Arabia and the Libyan Arab Jamehiriya, although the numbers of physicians involved were relatively small (21 and 18, respectively), *all* were born in countries other than these two countries of last permanent residence—in other words, only transient physicians migrated from these two countries to the United States in 1972.

The source on which table 1-15 is based indicates that, of the 7,143 physicians admitted as immigrants to the United States in 1972, 22 percent were not born in the country they claimed as the one of last permanent residence; for example, nearly a third of those coming from the Province of Taiwan were born elsewhere in Asia—primarily on the mainland of China; over half of those coming from Canada were born in an Asian country, about one-fifth in India alone; and over two-thirds of those coming from the United Kingdom were born in an Asian country, nearly half in India alone. [54] Thus, for a substantial fraction, their entry into the United States constituted at least a second migratory step, while for many others it may well have been a third or fourth step.

Another source, commenting on data concerning the immigration of

Table 1-15
Foreign Physicians Passing through Specified Countries (Way Stations) en Route to the United States[a]

Country of Last Permanent Residence but Not of Birth	*Number (1)*	*Percentage (2)*	*Country of Last Permanent Residence but Not of Birth*	*Number (1)*	*Percentage (2)*
Canada	339	77	Uganda	20	83
United Kingdom	314	86	Libyan Arab Rep.	18	100
China (Province of Taiwan)	155	33	Switzerland	18	72
Hong Kong	39	87	France	17	77
Israel	35	56	Japan	16	26
Germany, Fed. Rep. of	28	39	Italy	14	44
Lebanon	28	53	Australia	14	33
Saudi Arabia	21	100	Jamaica	13	72
Spain	20	34	Austria	12	80

Source: United States Bureau of Health Resources Development. Office of International Health Manpower Studies. *Foreign Medical Graduates and Physician Manpower in the United States*, DHEW Publication no. (HRA) 74-30 (Bethesda, Md.: U.S. Department of Health, Education, and Welfare, 1974).

Note: The countries selected were those where the number of physicians involved (column 1) was ten or more.

[a]Number in 1972 and as a percentage of the total admitted that year as immigrants to the United States from the specified country.

physicians to the United States in 1972, indicated that: neither the United Kingdom nor Canada is at present a substantial primary source of medical manpower for the United States; of the 439 immigrant physicians naming Canada as the country of last permanent residence, only 100 were born in Canada, the rest having been born in no fewer than 58 other countries; and of the 364 immigrant physicians naming the United Kingdom as the country of last permanent residence, only 50 were born in the United Kingdom, the rest having been born in 40 other countries. [20] The same source, commenting on data concerning the immigration of physicians from Canada and the United Kingdom to the United States during the years 1965-1972, stated that, during the first three years of that period, about two-fifths of immigrant physicians from Canada were born in Canada, but that in the three most recent years the proportion fell to one-fifth; comparable figures for the United Kingdom were four-fifths, later one-quarter.

Table 1-16 provides a reasonably clear picture of those countries whose native physicians use other countries (particularly those listed in the earlier table) as way stations. In terms of absolute numbers, the physicians who used way stations en route to the United States in 1972 were primarily those born in either India or the People's Republic of China. Proportionally, about one-third of the more than 3,000 physicians indicated in table 1-16 used way stations, the proportion for individual countries ranging from 22 to 78 percent.

On the basis of data appearing in two other sources, [20, 38] it was possible to ascertain that the following countries are most often used as way stations by physicians born elsewhere:

Country of Birth	*Main Way Stations*
China, People's Republic of	Province of Taiwan and Canada
Egypt	United Kingdom and Canada
India	Canada
United Kingdom	Canada
Poland	Italy and Canada
Romania	Canada and Italy
Cuba	Spain

Although no data are available on why certain physicians use certain countries as way stations to the United States, there appears to be some logic in the notion that physicians from Pakistan and India would follow the Commonwealth route through the United Kingdom and Canada; that physicians from Cuba (which had no formal diplomatic ties with the United States) would go to another Spanish-speaking country from which access to the United States would be facilitated; that physicians from Poland and Romania, because of their proximity to Italy, could avail themselves of the migrant-assisting voluntary agencies in Rome; and that physicians from the mainland of China would go through Taiwan because of the latter's close diplomatic ties with the United States at that time. Also noteworthy is the fact that, in many cases, the way station may also be the country of medical education.

The names of the United Kingdom, Hong Kong, Israel, Uganda, and Japan appear in both table 1-15 and table 1-16. These countries use way stations and are also used in this fashion. Other countries could be added to this group, although the numbers of physicians involved would be relatively small. Among the countries mentioned above, Israel acted as a way station for 35 of the physicians concerned; in turn, 11 physicians born in Israel entered the United States via other countries.

Outflow of FMGs from the United States

While immigration statistics, however crude, give some indication of the inflow of foreign physicians to the United States, corresponding emigration statistics are totally lacking. Consequently, it has not been possible to deter-

Table 1-16
Selected Countries of Origin of Physicians Who Use Way Stations en Route to the United States[a]

Country of Birth	*Total Number (1)*	*Number via Way Stations (2)*	*Percentage via Way Stations (2) ÷ (1) (3)*
India	1,802	392	22
China (excluding Taiwan)	274	214	78
Pakistan	260	130[b]	50
Egypt	115	58	50
Japan	76	31	41
Romania	47	28	60
United Kingdom	77	27	35
Poland	46	23	50
Indonesia	47	22	47
Burma	45	20	44
Cuba	73	19	26
Syrian Arab Rep.	29	13	45
Iraq	54	13	24
Czechoslovakia	34	12	35
Malaysia	21	12	57
Israel	38	11	29
Kenya	20	11	55
Hong Kong	16	10	62
Jordan	16	10	63
Haiti	28	8	29
Tanzania, United Rep.	21	7	33
Uganda	10	6	60

Source: Based on data in United States, Bureau of Health Resources Development office of International Health Manpower Studies, *Foreign Medical Graduates and Physician Manpower in the United States,* DHEW Publication no. (HRA) 74-30 (Bethesda, Md.: U.S. Department of Health, Education, and Welfare, 1974).

Notes: The countries selected were those where the number of physicians involved (column 2) was five or more.

[a]Total number of physicians, by country of birth, entering the United States as immigrants in 1972; and number and percentage entering the United States via countries other than country of birth.

[b]Includes Indians born in what are now Pakistan and Bangladesh.

mine the true magnitude of the net migration of foreign physicians to the United States. Estimates of the annual outflow of FMGs vary greatly, as do the methods used in making the estimates. The following method gives a rough indication, using data for the two-year period 1970–1972:

Stock of FMGs in 1970	57,217
Attrition (2 percent per annum)	2,288
	54,929
Inflow (2 years at 7,500 per annum)	15,000
	69,929
Stock in 1972	68,009
Outflow during the period	1,920
Rate of outflow per annum (1,920/15,000)	13%

The above rate of outflow—about 1,000 or 13 percent per annum—is somewhat lower than estimates arrived at by other means. Another method reported suggests that the return rate is considerably higher—about 1,500 or closer to 25 percent per annum. [13] The difference may well be due to the probability that the above-cited attrition rate of 2 percent per annum is too high for a young population of physicians (FMGs, being on average, much younger than USMGs).

The study on which the estimate of 25 percent is based used data from the annual census taken by the AMA's Physician Records Service. Through a computer-matching procedure, the entire population of FMGs in 1966 was compared with the entire population in 1968. Those FMGs who were recorded in both 1966 and 1968 had obviously not migrated, and thus were not included in the analysis. Those FMGs who were recorded in 1968 but not in 1966 were designated as increments to the physician population (inflow), while those who were recorded in 1966 but not in 1968 were designated as decrements (outflow).

Table 1-17, which comes from a report on the study, shows the relationship between inflow and outflow for the two-year period. Regarding the limitations of the data, the following observations can be made:

1. Both the inflow and the outflow may be underestimated, because in both cases the data fail to account for those FMGs not in the AMA's master file (the "underground"). However, this factor does not invalidate the indicated ratio of increments to decrements.

2. The outflow may be overestimated, because the data fail to distinguish between attrition through departure from the United States and attrition through death or retirement from the profession for other reasons.

3. The data on inflow as well as on outflow include FMGs born in the United States. However, given the likelihood that most U.S.-born FMGs will remain in the United States, the data on outflow presumably reflect a larger proportion of foreign-born FMGs than do the data on inflow. The net effect of this phenomenon is that, with respect to countries that provide medical education for many U.S. natives, the return rate (decrements) is underestimated. In the case of Spain, for example, it was shown earlier in

Table 1-17
Inflow (Increments) and Outflow (Decrements) of Foreign Physicians Who Entered the United States between Year End 1966 and 1968[a]

	Increments		*Decrements*		*Ratio of Increments to Decrements*
Region and Country	*Number (1)*	*Percentage (2)*	*Number (3)*	*Percentage (4)*	*(5)*
Asia	4,984	41	1,328	42	4:1
Philippines	1,724	14	419	13	4:1
India	1,073	9	333	10	3:1
Korea	559	5	59	2	9:1
Europe	3,167	26	999	31	3:1
Germany	529	4	211	7	3:1
Spain	367	3	34	1	11:1
United Kingdom	359	3	122	4	3:1
Latin America	2,401	20	297	9	8:1
Cuba	509	4	29	1	17:1
Colombia	415	3	46	1	9:1
Mexico	357	3	72	2	5:1
Rest of the world	1,520	13	548	17	3:1
Canada	1,025	9	485	15	2:1
Total	12,072	100	3,172	100	4:1

Source: I. Butter, "The Migratory Flow of Doctors to and from the United States," *Medical Care* 9(1971):17-31.

Note: Country designations are as indicated in the source.

[a] Regional totals and selected countries.

this chapter (table 1-7) that, of the FMGs from Spain who joined the pool of FMGs in the United States between the years 1966 and 1968, 35 percent were born in the United States. If that percentage were applied to the 367 FMGs from Spain who were indicated as increments in table 1-17, it would mean that only about 240 were foreign-born and that the ratio of increments to decrements with regard to Spain would be closer to 7:1 than to 11:1. It should be noted, however, that only a few countries—among them Spain, Italy, Mexico, Switzerland, and Canada—provide medical education for a substantial number of natives of the United States. The overall proportion of U.S. natives among the total FMGs in the United States is reported to be about 10 percent. If this is so, the overall ratio of increments to decrements with regard to alien FMGs, would be closer to 3:1 than to the 4:1 indicated in the table.

Reverting again to table 1-17, it is noteworthy that, with the exceptions of Spain (for the reason that 35 percent of FMGs were born in the United States), and Cuba (for political reasons), the tendency to remain in the United States is much greater among FMGs from Korea and Colombia than it is among those from India and the Philippines or among FMGs as a whole. Whereas the global average is one departure for every four FMGs entering, in the case of Colombia and Korea it is only one departure for every nine entering.

The findings from an eight-year follow-up study of a cohort of FMGs indicate that nearly 84 percent of those FMGs located in the United States in 1963 were still in the country in 1971. [25] Depending on the geographic area where the FMG had received training, the percentage remaining in the United States varied from over 73 percent for those graduating from Asian medical schools, to nearly 85 percent for those from Latin American schools and over 87 percent for those from European schools. On the assumption that those who were not located in the United States in 1971 had returned to their country of medical education, this would mean that 27 percent of the Asian graduates, 15 percent of the Latin American graduates, and 13 percent of the European graduates had returned to their country of medical education, the overall average of return being about 16 percent at the most. These figures indicate that Asian graduates manifest a considerably greater tendency to return than do Latin American and European graduates. The same study shows that among interns and residents the propensity to leave the United States is greater than it is among other categories of FMGs—about 26 percent leave as opposed to the overall average of 16 percent.

The findings from a similar study made of a much smaller cohort of FMGs in the United States, suggest that, with few exceptions, donor countries permanently lose between two-thirds and three-quarters of those of their medical graduates who go to the United States for further study or for work. [47] Of those who do not remain in the United States, the majority return to their country of medical education. A few go to other countries. This study also suggests that, within a seven-year period, one out of six foreign-trained interns and residents in the United States can be expected to leave the United States and then return at a later date. The study further suggests that, of those FMGs who leave the United States, the majority are under 35 years of age. After leaving the United States they tend to gravitate toward teaching, research, and full-time hospital positions. A small proportion enter private practice, mainly in major cities and in relatively esoteric fields, such as cardiology or endocrinology.

Of a total of 760 respondents to a questionnaire sent in 1974 to 2,270 Iranian physicians listed by the AMA as residing in the United States in 1973, 249 (35 percent) indicated they definitely would not return to Iran,

372 (52 percent) indicated that they planned to return to Iran in the next five years, and 12 percent indicated that they had not yet made a definite decision. [43] Of those who were undergoing specialty training, 84 percent expressed an intention to return to Iran, as opposed to 35 percent of those not in training, the latter figure representing essentially an older population of physicians. Those physicians who had previously practiced in Iran were significantly more likely to be planning to return to Iran within the subsequent five years—61 percent of those who had practiced in Iran, as opposed to 41 percent of those who had not, indicated their intention to return to Iran. Of those Iranian physicians who had received their basic medical education in Iran, 56 percent definitely planned to return to Iran, as opposed to only 27 percent of those who had received such education outside Iran. For those physicians who were planning to return within the next five years, a university position was by far the most desired position, while the least desirable position was government service.

A study that analyzed the whereabouts of 1,436 physicians who had graduated from Colombian medical schools before 1970 and who had migrated to the United States showed that, as of 21 September 1973, 1,023 (71 percent) were still in the United States, 314 (22 percent) were in Colombia, and 99 (7 percent) could not be traced. [72] The return rates, by year of the physicians' graduation, are interesting to note (table 1-18).

The study also found that most Colombian physicians migrated to the United States within five years of graduation from medical school, and that those who returned to Colombia within the same five-year period did not, for the most part, remigrate to the United States. The remainder of those who returned to Colombia did so within five to ten years of graduation, and a small proportion of them remigrated to the United States. Remigration to

Table 1-18
Return Rate for Physicians Educated in Colombia, by Year of Graduation

Year of Graduation	*Number of Migrants to United States*	*Located in Colombia in September 1973*	
		Number	*Percentage*
Before 1940	37	28	76
1940-1944	48	34	71
1945-1949	77	38	49
1950-1954	172	51	30
1955-1959	317	60	19
1960-1964	459	82	18
1965-1969	326	21	6
Total	1,436	314	22

Table 1–19
Emigration of American Physicians: Number Found to Be in Specified Countries, and Number Entering Canada and New Zealand as Immigrants

Year	*Found in United Kingdom (1)*	*Found in Federal Republic of Germany (2)*	*Found in Ethiopia (3)*	*Found in Australia (4)*	*Found in Japan (5)*	*Found in Austria (6)*	*Found in Niger (7)*	*Found in Singapore (8)*	*Found in Sweden (9)*	*Found in Laos (10)*	*Entering New Zealand (11)*	*Entering Canada (12)*
1961					12							
1962					16							97
1963					8							143
1964					10							60
1965					16							42
1966	172			21	16	7						58
1967					14	4	2		1			
1968					14	5					6	
1969					9	7					20	
1970	170				13					7	13	
1971		49	28									
1972												
1973								1				115
1974												116

Source: World Health Organization, ''Multinational Study of the International Migration of Physicians and Nurses: Statistical Enquiry'' (unpublished information).

Note: Column 3 includes dentists.

the United States represented about one out of every six returnees, and one out of every thirty-four migrants.

Outflow of American Physicians from the United States

Only about 1,300 physicians of American nationality (that is, citizens of the United States) were traced by a WHO study as being abroad in the early 1970s. [68] This number is equivalent to less than 0.5 percent of the active population of physicians in the United States in 1974. Considering that there were about 69,000 foreign-born and foreign-trained physicians in the United States in 1974, one can say that for every 53 such physicians in the United States, one American physician was found abroad. The location of these physicians is shown in table 1-19. Most are in English-speaking countries: About 100 per year have been entering Canada in recent years, and 170 were reported to be in the United Kingdom in 1970. There appears to be no published information on either the general characteristics of American physicians abroad or on their rate of return to the United States.

2 Characteristics and Career Patterns of FMGs

Around 1970 FMGs in the United States constituted an essentially younger population than did USMGs. The youngest group consisted largely of Asians, the oldest largely of Europeans. About 40 percent of FMGs had graduated between the years 1960 and 1970. The proportion of women was over twice as large among FMGs as among USMGs. Nearly a third of the FMGs from the Philippines were women, matching the proportion of women in the pool of physicians in the Philippines.

Regarding modes and areas of practice, both FMGs and USMGs were largely engaged in direct patient care, with the difference that proportionally more FMGs than USMGs functioned in a hospital setting and more were interns, residents, and full-time hospital staff. FMGs were more inclined toward research and less toward administration. About equal proportions of FMGs and USMGs were engaged in medical teaching. Over two-thirds of FMGs were concentrated in a group of eight specialties, with the highest proportions in general practice, internal medicine, general surgery, and psychiatry. There appears to be a shift away from general practice and psychiatry, and a greater movement toward internal medicine and general surgery.

Most FMGs decided to go to the United States before or soon after completing undergraduate studies, but decided to remain in the United States only after a stay in the country. Those who left the United States tended to return to their country of medical education, most commonly to teach medicine. The more advanced the FMG was in his training, the greater his tendency to remain in the United States. Older FMGs were more likely than younger ones to remain. Of those remaining, most were licensed to practice medicine in the United States.

A special category of FMG is composed of foreign physicians who achieved immigrant status. A cohort of such physicians is described in terms of their experiences with respect to the ECFMG examination, licensure, and areas and modes of practice. Another special category of FMGs is the unlicensed contingent, whose number is thought to be large and many of whom are providing direct patient care. A sample of this group is described in terms of their specialty training and work experience prior to their entry to the United States.

FMGs by Age

In 1970, FMGs in the United States constituted an essentially young population, with nearly one-half under 40 years of age and an average age of 43 years. By comparison, USMGs represented a somewhat older population and graduates of Canadian schools an even older one (table 2-1).

The oldest group of FMGs consisted largely of Europeans, who arrived in the United States in two phases: (1) during the 1930s, primarily from Germany, and in the late 1930s also from other parts of war-torn Europe; and (2) during the late 1940s, as part of a general exodus from countries ravaged by the war. The fact that the group of graduates from schools in Belgium, Italy, Spain, and Switzerland contained a substantial proportion of natives of the United States obscures the picture with regard to nationals of those countries, whose age structure may actually have been similar to that of graduates from other European countries.

About 27 percent of the FMGs from European countries (including the four countries mentioned above) were at least 60 years old. The source on which table 2-1 is based indicates that countries having the largest propor-

Table 2-1
Age Distribution of Medical Graduates in the United States, by Geographic Area of Graduation, 1970

Geographic Area of Graduation	*Age in Years*				
	All (Percentage)	*Under 40 (Percentage)*	*40-59 (Percentage)*	*60 and Over (Percentage)*	*Number*
Asia	100	75	24	1	21,875
Oceania	100	59	38	3	404
Latin America (excluding Cuba)	100	58	40	2	7,172
Africa	100	58	41		1,125
Italy, Spain, Switzerland, and Belgium	100	30	53	16	8,030
Other Europe	100	22	46	32	15,845
Cuba	100	7	78	15	2,757
All FMGs	100	47	40	13	57,217
USMGs	100	37	42	21	270,637
Canadian MGs	100	31	43	26	6,174

Source: American Medical Association, Center for Health Services Research and Development, *Foreign Medical Graduates in the United States, 1970,* ed. J.N. Haug and B.C. Martin (Chicago: American Medical Association, 1971).

tion of their graduates in that age group were Austria (61 percent), the German Democratic Republic (83 percent), and the USSR (63 percent). [3] Others having a relatively large proportion were Czechoslovakia (47 percent), France (40 percent), Hungary (44 percent), and Poland (43 percent). Graduates from the socialist countries represented almost exclusively those who migrated before World War II, except for those migrating from Hungary after 1956 and from Czechoslovakia after 1968. The age distribution of FMGs from the latter, as shown in table 2-2, illustrates the point that FMGs from the socialist countries are as a whole only of historical importance, since the outflow from those countries has virtually stopped.

The youngest group of FMGs in 1970 consisted largely of Asians, of whom 75 percent were under 40 years of age and only 1 percent over 60 years. Typically, the average age of graduates from the Philippines was 36 years, and that of graduates from India 33 years, compared to an average age of 43 years for all FMGs. Major donor countries whose graduates in the United States were mostly under 40 years of age included Argentina (68 percent), Belgium (52 percent), Colombia (69 percent), India (88 percent), Iran (76 percent), Japan (63 percent), Lebanon (47 percent), Pakistan (93 per-

Table 2-2
Foreign Medical Graduates in the United States from Czechoslovakia and Hungary

Age in 1970	*Number from Czechoslovakia*	*Number from Hungary*
< 30	20	1
30-34	27	13
35-39	45	10
40-44	64[a]	119
45-49	40	122[a]
50-54	53	94
55-59	95	122[b]
60-64	134[b]	111
65-69	70	84
70-74	165	92
≥ 75	41	94
Percentage over retirement age	27%	31%

[a] Illustrates the peak in the outflow from Eastern European countries generally before World War II.

[b] Reflects a peak in outflow from Hungary and Czechoslovakia as a result of political events in 1956 and 1968, respectively.

cent), Peru (57 percent), Philippines (76 percent), Republic of Korea (82 percent), Spain (53 percent), Taiwan (86 percent), Thailand (96 percent), and Egypt (61 percent). Except for the cases of Belgium and Spain, many of whose graduates were U.S. natives, this phenomenon reflects the United States' abandonment in 1965 of the national-origins quotas, a move that facilitated the inflow from developing countries of thousands of physicians, including many young graduates. The distorted age distribution of graduates from Cuba, shown in table 2-1, reflects a mass exodus of established physicians from that country in the 1950s.

FMGs by Year of Graduation

Closely linked to the age distribution of FMGs in the United States is their distribution by year of graduation. The study cited previously indicates that approximately 40 percent of FMGs in the United States in 1970 graduated between 1960 and 1970. [3] This high percentage reflects mainly the large inflow of new graduates from Asian medical schools. The percentage distribution of FMGs in 1970, by year of graduation, was as follows:

Year	*Percentage*	*Year*	*Percentage*
Before 1920	1	1945–1949	7
1920–1924	2	1950–1954	14
1925–1929	2	1955–1959	18
1930–1934	3	1960–1964	23
1935–1939	6	1965–1969	19
1940–1944	5		

Those graduating before 1930 were mainly from Austria, Cuba, Czechoslovakia, the German Democratic Republic, Hungary, Italy, Poland, and the USSR. For certain donor countries, and even for certain groups of donor countries, those physicians who qualified during a particular decade feature more prominently in the FMG statistics than do those qualifying during other decades. The following table shows a number of countries grouped according to the decade in which the largest proportion of their graduates found in the United States had graduated:

Decade	*Country*	*Decade*	*Country*
1920–1929	German Democratic Republic	1935–1944	Hungary USSR
1930–1939	Austria France Poland	1940–1949	China (excluding Taiwan)

Decade	*Country*	*Decade*	*Country*
1945–1954	Cuba Federal Republic of Germany Romania	1955–1964 (cont'd)	Iraq Israel Japan Mexico Spain Switzerland
1950–1959	Dominican Republic Greece Italy Netherlands Poland Turkey United Kingdom Yugoslavia	1960–1970	India Iran Lebanon Pakistan Philippines Republic of Korea China (Taiwan only) Thailand Venezuela
1955–1964	Argentina Colombia Egypt Haiti		

The distributions of FMGs by age and by year of graduation are not only linked to each other, but also reflect the precursors and aftermaths of global conflicts and/or political events in individual countries. They also reflect changes in the admission laws of the United States.

FMGs by Sex

In 1970 females represented 15 percent of the pool of FMGs in the United States, compared with 13 percent in 1963. The proportion of women among FMGs was over twice as large as that among either USMGs or the graduates of Canadian medical schools who were in the pool of physicians in the United States at the time, the proportions being respectively 15, 6, and 7 percent.

Female FMGs constituted at least 20 percent of all FMGs from the following countries: the Philippines (31 percent); China, Poland, Thailand, and the USSR (each with 27 percent); Yugoslavia (24 percent); Romania (22 percent); and India and the Republic of Korea (each with 21 percent). [3]

It is interesting to compare the proportion of female FMGs from individual countries of graduation, with the proportion of females in the pool of physicians in each respective country (table 2–3). Among the Asian countries listed, these proportions were equal in the case of the Philippines and Thailand. For the Republic of Korea and Indonesia the proportions in each case were highly disparate, but in opposite senses: Whereas there were proportionally more females among Indonesia's domestic pool of physi-

Table 2-3
Percentage of Females among Foreign Medical Graduates in the United States in 1970, Compared with Percentage of Females in the Pool of Physicians in the Country of Graduation for the Year Specified

	Percentage of Females	
Country of Graduation	*Among Pool of Physicians in Country of Graduation (1)*	*Among Pool of FMGs in USA (2)*
Philippines	31 (1973)	31
Thailand	26 (1968)	27
Republic of Korea	16 (1968)	21
Indonesia	15 (1973)	9
Egypt	14 (1970)	7
Argentina	7 (1960)	14
Brazil	10 (1970)	9
Colombia	2 (1965)	3
Canada	10 (1971)	6
Austria	21 (1971)	19
Czechoslovakia	42 (1970)	16
Poland	51 (1970)	27
Federal Republic of Germany	25 (1970)	19
Belgium	10 (1970)	7
Spain	4 (1970)	9
Switzerland	14 (1970)	8

Sources (column 1): for Colombia, R. Paredes-Maurique and C. Agualimpia, *Study of Human Resources for Health and Medical Education in Colombia: Methods and Results*, (Bogota: Ministry of Public Health and Colombian Association of Medical Faculties, 1972); for other countries, World Health Organization, *World Health Statistics' Annual 1972*, vol. 3 (Geneva: World Health Organization, 1974); (column 2): American Medical Association, Center for Health Services Research and Development, *Foreign Medical Graduates in the United States, 1970*, ed. J.N. Haug and B.C. Martin (Chicago: American Medical Association, 1971).

cians than among its emigrant physicians, the reverse was so in the case of the Republic of Korea. The question arises as to what forces acting on women exclusively resulted in the greater tendency of Korea's female physicians to leave the country, and of Indonesia's to remain at home. Egypt's pattern was similar to that of Indonesia. Both are Moslem countries, where perhaps female physicians, more than male physicians, are called on to cater to the health-care needs of women. The proportion of women among FMGs from Latin America was probably equal to that among domestic stock, although the table suggests otherwise—most probably because, in the case of Argentina and Colombia, information on domestic stock was much older than that on FMGs. As for Canada's medical graduates, fewer females migrated than males. With regard to European countries, a distinction must be made between new and old cohorts, the latter reflecting the situation in the home country during an earlier era. As for those European countries that are predominantly exporters of medical education to the United States, the picture may be blurred by the probability that, of the FMGs from those countries, the U.S.-born contingent was more heavily represented by males than was the native contingent.

Within the FMG pool as a whole in 1970, the females tended to be younger than the males: 42 percent of the females, as opposed to 28 percent of the males, were under 35 years of age, while the respective proportions for those under 30 years of age were 16 and 8 percent. The relatively younger age of the female contingent may be a result of the fact that, in recent years, the largest numbers of FMGs were from countries whose physicians were largely young and whose proportion of female physicians was relatively high—for example, in the Philippines and Thailand.

Modes of Practice of FMGs

Around 1970 most FMGs were engaged in direct patient care, most often in a hospital setting. Those not directly involved in patient care tended more toward research than toward other areas of professional activity. Table 2-4 shows some interesting similarities and contrasts between FMGs and USMGs regarding modes of practice. As one would expect, very high and almost equal proportions of each were engaged in direct patient care, the difference being that: (1) proportionately more of all FMGs than of all USMGs functioned in a hospital setting; and (2) within the hospital setting, proportionately more of all FMGs than of all USMGs were interns, residents, and full-time staff; about 48 percent of all FMGs were trainees and full-time staff, compared with only 24 percent of all USMGs.

The relatively high proportion of FMGs who were trainees was reflected, in turn, in the substantially smaller proportion of FMGs who managed to have some private practice in a hospital setting; 19 percent of USMG time was spent in private practice in a hospital setting, compared with only 12 percent of FMG time. In either case, the extent to which such practice was conducted by physicians who had a regular office-based practice outside the hospital was not indicated. In both cases, about two-and-a-half times as much time was spent in private practice in an office setting, as in a hospital setting.

As for other modes of practice, proportionately more of the FMGs than of the USMGs tended toward research activities. That the proportion

Table 2-4
Modes of Practice of Foreign Medical Graduates, Compared with Those of United States Medical Graduates, 1973

	USMGs		*FMGs*	
Mode of Practice	*Number (1)*	*Percentage (2)*	*Number (3)*	*Percentage (4)*
All modes of practice	261,858	100	62,509	100
All direct patient care	237,920	91	57,337	92
All private practice	174,165	66	27,270	44
Private practice in office setting	124,282	47	19,694	31
Private prac- in hospital setting	49,883	19	7,576	12
Interns and residents	39,059	15	19,193	31
Full-time hospital staff	24,696	10	10,874	17
Medical teaching	4,943	2	1,240	2
Administration	10,604	4	1,355	2
Research	6,246	2	2,086	3
Other modes of practice	2,145	1	491	1

Source: A. Lowin, *FMGs? An Evaluation of Policy-Related Research,* Prepared for the National Science Foundation, Washington, D.C., NSF-C814 (Minneapolis: Inter Study, 1975).

Notes: Figures exclude physicians not classified by mode of practice, those who are inactive, and those whose address is unknown. All figures relating to both modes of private practice represent equivalents based on patient visits per week.

of each was very low, however, may well be due to the fact that, for at least the past decade, American medical schools have focused largely on the production of research workers who were not necessarily physicians (a factor that is discussed more fully in chapter 3). Presumably, therefore, most health research was being undertaken by individuals trained exclusively for that purpose. In the area of administration, the proportion of USMGs was twice that of FMGs. With respect to medical teaching and unspecified modes of practice, the proportions were about equal.

While this study shows a static picture of the modes of practice of physicians in 1973, another study shows their mobility, but with respect to FMGs only. The unit of observation was a cohort of 32,699 FMGs—all those known to be in the United States in 1963. The modes of practice of the cohort were observed at two points in time, 1963 and 1971, representing an interval of eight years. Tables 2-5 and 2-6, which come from a report of that study, [25] indicate the following:

1. Of all FMGs in the United States in 1963, over half were in office-based practice in the United States in 1971. Whereas office-based practice occupied 14,401 or 44 percent of the cohort in 1963, it occupied 16,971 or 52 percent in 1971—a rise of 8 percent. The rise would have been higher except for the fact that nearly one-quarter of those FMGs who were in office-based practice in 1963 had moved elsewhere by 1971. Many went into hospital settings, others into teaching, administration, and research. Quite a few became inactive or returned to their homelands.
2. Of the three groups of FMGs in hospital practice in 1963 (interns, residents, and full-time hospital staff), residents showed the greatest tendency to move to office-based practice. Thus, nearly 38 percent of the residents, as opposed to nearly 34 percent of the full-time staff and 29 percent of the interns, had moved to office-based practice. This would appear to reflect a normal move upward in the career ladder.
3. Of the 778 FMGs in medical teaching posts in 1963, nearly one-third had moved to office-based practice by 1971. Thus for FMGs, teaching posts, like internships, residencies, and full-time hospital-staff appointments, acted as a channel to office-based practice.
4. In terms of professional mobility:
   a. Those already in office-based practice in 1963 were the least mobile, with only 24 percent moving out and, of these, only one-third going into other modes of practice, mainly into full-time hospital-staff positions.
   b. Those in administration were the next least mobile group, with 42 percent remaining in administration, about 22 percent moving into office-based practice, and 10 percent moving into full-time hospital-staff positions.
   c. Those in internship and residency positions were, as would be expected, the most mobile, with 313 (only about 3 percent) remaining in such positions by 1971. It is surprising that even that large a number remained, an indication that there exists a group of FMGs who regard internship and residency as a way of life.
   d. Those in medical teaching were the next most mobile, with less than 18 percent remaining in medical training and, of the remainder, about one-third moving into office-based practice and one-fifth into research.

Table 2–5
Activities of Foreign Medical Graduates in the United States in 1963, Compared with Their Activities in 1971, in Absolute Numbers

		1971 Distribution of 1963 FMG Population by Activity											
Activity	*1963 Distribution of FMG Population*	*Office-Based Practice*	*Interns*	*Residents*	*Hospital Physician Staff*	*Medical Teaching*	*Adminis-tration*	*Research*	*Other*[a]	*Not Classified*	*Inactive*	*Address Unknown*	*Not on 1971 Record*
Total	32,699	16,971	13	414	5,036	560	865	798	289	449	1,465	475	5,364
Office based practice	14,401	10,947	0	55	775	70	169	79	79	102	718	113	1,294
Interns	2,141	626	2	149	529	34	18	59	26	116	37	80	465
Residents	7,800	2,942	10	152	1,650	145	117	180	72	138	98	147	2,149
Hospital physician staff	4,388	1,481	1	26	1,553	95	254	79	42	52	202	72	531
Medical teaching	778	258	0	2	64	137	65	157	6	4	16	3	66
Administration	178	40	0	0	18	3	75	2	4	0	20	1	15
Research	901	225	0	13	131	37	48	190	9	9	21	9	209
Classification unknown[b]	1,016	299	0	5	226	31	108	32	46	23	56	15	175
Inactive	1,096	153	0	12	90	8	11	20	5	5	297	35	460
Address unknown[c]	0	0	0	0	0	0	0	0	0	0	0	0	0

Source: J.N. Haug and R. Stevens, "Foreign Medical Graduates in the United States in 1963 and 1971: A Cohort Study," *Inquiry* 10(1973):26–32.

[a] This activity classification did not exist in 1963.

[b] Since classification criteria were modified in 1968 based on the Reclassification of Physicians, classification by activity for 1963 is not available for these physicians. See American Medical Association, *Reclassification of Physicians* (Chicago: American Medical Association, 1971).

[c] Those with address unknown were distributed by activity for 1963.

Table 2–6
Activities of Foreign Medical Graduates in the United States in 1963, Compared with Their Activities in 1971, in Percentages

		1971 Distribution of 1963 FMG Population by Activity (Percentages)											
Activity	*1963 Distribution of FMG Population*	*Office-Based Practice*	*Interns*	*Residents*	*Hospital Physician Staff*	*Medical Teaching*	*Adminis-tration*	*Research*	*Other*[a]	*Not Classified*	*Inactive*	*Address Unknown*	*Not on 1971 Record*
Total	100.0	51.9	0.0	1.3	15.4	1.7	2.6	2.4	0.9	1.4	4.5	1.5	16.4
Office based practice	100.0	76.0	0.0	0.4	5.4	0.5	1.2	0.5	0.5	0.7	5.0	0.8	9.0
Interns	100.0	29.2	0.1	7.0	24.7	1.6	0.8	2.8	1.2	5.4	1.7	3.7	21.7
Residents	100.0	37.7	0.1	1.9	21.2	1.9	1.5	2.3	0.9	1.8	1.3	1.9	27.6
Hospital physician staff	100.0	33.8	0.0	0.6	35.4	2.1	5.8	1.8	1.0	1.2	4.6	1.6	12.1
Medical teaching	100.0	33.2	0.0	0.3	8.2	17.6	8.4	20.2	0.8	0.5	2.1	0.4	8.5
Administration	100.0	22.5	0.0	0.0	10.1	1.7	42.1	1.1	2.2	0.0	11.2	0.6	8.4
Research	100.0	25.0	0.0	1.4	14.5	4.1	5.3	21.1	1.0	1.0	2.3	1.0	23.2
Classification unknown[b]	100.0	29.4	0.0	0.5	22.2	3.1	10.6	3.1	4.5	2.3	5.5	1.5	17.2
Inactive	100.0	14.0	0.0	1.1	8.2	0.8	1.0	1.8	0.5	0.5	27.1	3.2	42.0
Address unknown[c]	0.0	—	—	—	—	—	—	—	—	—	—	—	—

Source: J.N. Haug and R. Stevens, "Foreign Medical Graduates in the United States in 1963 and 1971: A Cohort Study," *Inquiry* 10(1973):26–32.

[a] This activity classification did not exist in 1963.

[b] Since classification criteria were modified in 1968 based on the Reclassification of Physicians, classification by activity for 1963 is not available for these physicians. See American Medical Association, *Reclassification of Physicians* (Chicago, American Medical Association, 1971).

[c] Those with address unknown were distributed by activity for 1963.

e. Those in research were also quite mobile, with about 21 percent remaining in research, 25 percent moving to office-based practice, and less than 15 percent moving to full-time hospital-staff positions.

5. In general, for nearly 60 percent of the cohort of FMGs, either their mode of practice or their status was different in 1971 from what it was in 1963.
6. Over 80 percent of the FMGs located in the United States in 1963 were still there in 1971. For those who were interns and residents, the proportion was 74 percent, most of whom were in apparently permanent positions.

Specialties of FMGs

Although all specialties in the United States attracted a certain number of FMGs, some appeared to have a much greater drawing power than others. Table 2-7, which reflects data from a study sponsored by the AMA, [3] indicates the following:

1. In 1970, over two-thirds of all FMGs were concentrated in a group of eight out of thirty-four specified specialties. The largest proportion, nearly 12 percent, were in general practice, followed by internal medicine, general surgery, psychiatry, pediatrics, anesthesiology, pathology, and obstetrics and gynecology; in that order.
2. By comparison, physicians trained in the United States and Canada manifested a similar pattern, except that anesthesiology and pathology were replaced by radiology, ophthalmology, and orthopedic surgery, fields with considerably lower FMG participation.
3. With respect to groups of specialties, proportionally more of those graduating in the United States and Canada than of those graduating elsewhere tended toward surgical specialties. The same was true for general practice. With respect to medical specialties, the proportions were almost equal. Specialties other than medical and surgical drew a substantially higher proportion of FMGs—over 40 percent compared with 26 percent for other physicians. This is attributable to the relatively high proportions of FMGs specializing in psychiatry, anesthesiology, and pathology.

Another study, which examined the specialty distribution of individual cohorts of FMGs who had achieved immigrant status in the United States during specified years, shows quite clearly how their pattern of distribution has been changing over the years. Table 2-8, which comes from a report of that study, indicates a striking trend away from general practice and psy-

Table 2-7
Physicians in the United States in 1970: Proportions in Each Specialty, by Country of Graduation
(percent)

Specialty	*Graduated in United States or Canada (N = 256,703)*	*Graduated Elsewhere (N = 54,142)*
General practice	19.9	12.4
Medical specialties	25.0	24.0
Allergology	0.5	0.3
Cardiovascular diseases	2.0	2.3
Dermatology	1.4	0.7
Gastroenterology	0.6	0.7
Internal medicine	13.8	11.7
Pediatrics	5.6	6.5
Pediatric allergology	0.1	0.1
Pediatric cardiology	0.1	0.3
Pulmonary diseases	0.6	1.1
Surgical specialties	28.6	23.0
General surgery	9.5	9.7
Neurological surgery	0.8	0.7
Obstetrics and gynecology	6.1	5.6
Ophthalmology	3.5	1.4
Orthopedic surgery	3.4	1.6
Otolaryngology	1.8	1.1
Plastic surgery	0.5	0.3
Colonic/rectal surgery	0.2	0.1
Thoracic surgery	0.5	0.6
Urology	1.9	1.3
Other specialties	23.3	40.5
Aviation medicine	0.4	0.0[a]
Anesthesiology	2.9	6.1
Child psychiatry	0.6	0.7
Diagnostic roentgenology	0.6	0.6
Forensic pathology	0.0[a]	0.0
Neurology	0.9	1.1
Occupational medicine	0.9	0.3
Psychiatry	6.2	9.2
Pathology	2.7	5.7
General preventive medicine	0.5	0.1
Physical medicine and rehabilitation	0.1	0.9
Public health	1.0	0.4
Radiology	3.5	2.5
Therapeutic radiology	0.2	0.3
Other specialties	1.7	4.5
Unspecified	3.3	7.1

Source: Based on data in American Medical Association, Center for Health Services Research and Development, *Foreign Medical Graduates in the United States, 1970,* ed. J.N. Haug and B.C. Martin (Chicago: American Medical Association, 1971).

Note: Totals on which percentages are based exclude physicians not classified, inactive physicians, and those whose address is unknown.

[a] 0.0 = less than 0.05.

chiatry, and an equally striking trend toward internal medicine and general surgery. [32] With regard to anesthesiology and pathology, there was a slight downward movement in the former and an even slighter upward movement in the latter. The striking changes with respect to general practice, psychiatry, internal medicine, and general surgery give rise to several questions, such as: Are fewer FMGs going into general practice and psychiatry because more USMGs are beginning to take an interest in these areas of work? Is the opposite true with respect to general surgery and internal medicine? (Some insight into these two questions may be gained from chapter 4, which provides, among other things, an analysis of the relationship between the specialties chosen by USMGs and the manner in which the FMGs filled the remaining gaps.) What is the relationship between the "self-designated" specialty of the FMG and the actual specialty in which he is engaged? Does the changing composition of the FMG pool by area of origin, after 1965, have anything to do with changes in the specialty distribution of the pool—in other words, would Asian FMGs be more likely than European and/or Latin American FMGs to choose general surgery and internal medicine, and less likely to choose general practice and psychiatry? (The answer to this last question could be of particular interest to donor countries.) Does the changing composition of the FMG pool by age have a bearing on specialty distribution?

FMGs Who Leave and Those Who Stay in the United States

Although studies such as those previously cited give a good indication of the career patterns of FMGs at particular points or intervals of time, they shed light neither on the paths taken by FMGs from the point of their entry into the American medical system, nor on the ways in which these paths differ from those taken by USFMGs. Up to now, little has been published on the second aspect; but the first has been at least partly covered by a longitudinal study of all FMGs appointed to graduate training positions in hospitals in Connecticut in 1964. [47]

The majority of the FMGs studied decided to go to the United States either while still undergraduates or soon after graduation. A few had made the decision even before entering medical school. A little over one-third had considered going to countries other than the United States, usually the United Kingdom or Canada. The reasons for coming to the United States varied, but in general it appears that the decision to migrate reflected not so much the FMG's desire to obtain the best possible training, as it did his judgment of how best to advance his medical career.

The majority of FMGs who decided to stay in the United States made

Table 2-8
Percentage Distribution, by Self-Designated Specialty, of Cohorts of Foreign Physicians Admitted as Immigrants to the United States during Specified Years

	Years				
Specialty	*1961–1965 (%)*	*1966–1967 (%)*	*1968–1969 (%)*	*1970–1971 (%)*	*Total (%)*
General practice	9	8	7	3	7
Internal medicine	12	13	14	18	14
Pediatrics	6	7	9	8	7
Other medical specialties	6	5	4	4	5
General surgery	9	10	12	16	11
Obstetrics/ gynecology	6	6	8	8	7
Other surgical specialties	10	10	8	8	9
Anesthesiology	8	9	9	8	9
Psychiatry	13	11	8	7	10
Pathology	7	7	8	8	7
Other specialties	14	14	14	12	13
Total	100	100	100	100	100
Number: Total	1,945	1,493	1,745	1,701	6,884
Specialty unspecified	12	32	75	267	386

Source: J.C. Kleinman, R.J. Weiss, and D.S. Felsenthal, "Immigrant Physicians. Results of a Cohort Study." *Inquiry* 12(1975):193-203.

Note: Only those immigrant physicians matched to the AMA file are included in this table.

this decision only after the attractions of the United States had made themselves felt and/or after being offered posts. Only 21 percent claimed that when they first arrived they already intended to remain in the country; 67 percent actually did remain, or at least were still there in 1971, seven years after the first point at which they were observed. Another 4 percent were in Canada. Those who left the United States tended to return to their countries of medical education.

Neither the size nor type of hospital in which the physician undertook his training in 1964, nor the size of community in which the hospital was situated, appeared to play an important role in the decision to leave or to remain in the United States. The more advanced the physician was in his training in 1971, the greater was his tendency to remain in the United States: About 10 percent more of the residents than of the interns remained.

In relation to others in their age group, the older physicians (those over 35 years of age in 1964) showed a greater tendency to remain in the United States than did the younger ones: Whereas 92 percent of the former stayed, only 68 percent of the latter did so (table 2-9). On the whole, the older physicians tended to have been in the United States for some time and to have moved from one training position to another, perhaps because of a failure to become licensed. With regard to all the members of the study group found abroad in 1971, 97 percent were then less than 43 years old and thus had considerable time ahead in which to realize their potential. Of the group remaining in the United States, 83 percent were less than 43 years old.

With respect to the modes of practice in 1971 for those on whom information was available (table 2-10), nearly half of the physicians remaining in the United States were in salaried positions—38 percent as full-time hospital staff and 10 percent in teaching and research. Over one-third were in private practice. Surprisingly, about 15 percent were still in training. One of the reasons put forward for the "eternal-intern syndrome" is that, for whatever reason, a foreign physician on an exchange visitor's visa either does not dare or does not wish to apply for a change of visa status; so long as he remains as an exchange visitor, he is not eligible to apply for a license to practice in the United States. Thus many foreign physicians remain in jobs that do not require a license. Among those physicians who left the United States the proportion going into private practice was substantially smaller than among their colleagues who remained; on the other hand, the proportion going into teaching and research was three times higher. The desire to teach appeared to be the strongest single factor encouraging physicians to return home. Whether opportunities for teaching in the United States were available to them was not investigated. On the whole, the returnees tended to work in major cities and in relatively esoteric fields, such as cardiology and endocrinology. It would appear, according to the report of the authors of this study, that the United States is training foreign graduates primarily for hospital work in the United States, and secondarily for elite positions abroad. This notion is further confirmed by the data in tables 2-7 and 2-8.

The study also indicated that, of the 183 FMGs on whom citizenship information was available, about one-fifth had become American citizens between their year of graduation and 1971. The proportions acquiring citizenship varied from one country of graduation to another, with graduates of India and the Philippines reflecting very low percentages, 4 and 8 percent respectively. The explanation appears to be that a relatively high proportion of Indians and Filipinos in the group had entered as exchange visitors, and had either kept this status or had not, at the time, met the five-year residence requirement that immigrants must fulfill before applying for American citizenship.

With regard to licensing, there was a marked difference between those

Table 2-9
Percentage Distribution (and Number) of a Cohort of Foreign Medical Graduates, by Location in 1971 and Age in 1964

	Location in 1971			
Age in 1964	*United States (%) (Number)*	*Elsewhere (%) (Number)*	*Total (%) (Number)*	*Unknown (Number)*
20–25	14 (30)	20 (17)	16 (47)	(5)
26–30	47 (101)	51 (44)	48 (145)	(7)
31–35	22 (46)	26 (22)	23 (68)	(5)
36+	17 (37)	3 (3)	13 (40)	(2)
Total	100 (214)	100 (86)	100 (300)	(19)

Source: Based on data in R.A. Stevens, L.W. Goodman, and S.S. Mick, "What Happens to Foreign-Trained Doctors Who Come to the United States," *Inquiry* 11(1974):112–124.

Table 2-10
Percentage Distribution (and Number) of a Cohort of Foreign Medical Graduates, by Mode of Medical Practice and Location in 1971

	Location in 1971			
Mode of Medical Practice in 1971	*United States (%) (Number)*	*Elsewhere (%) (Number)*	*Total (%) (Number)*	*Unknown (Number)*
Private practice	37 (76)	30 (17)	35 (93)	(0)
Full-time hospital	38 (79)	35 (20)	38 (99)	(0)
Teaching/research	10 (20)	30 (17)	14 (37)	(0)
Training	15 (30)	5 (3)	13 (33)	(0)
Total	100 (205)	100 (57)	100 (262)	
Other and unknown	(9)	(29)	(38)	(19)

Source: Based on data in R.A. Stevens, L.W. Goodman, and S.S. Mick, "What Happens to Foreign-Trained Doctors Who Come to the United States," *Inquiry* 11(1974):112–124.

who remained in the United States and those who left. Of those who remained and on whom information was available, 88 percent held a license to practice in the United States. Only six of those abroad held such a license. This finding would appear to confirm the suggestion made earlier in this book that the holding of a license is a good indication of intent to remain in the United States.

The Immigrant FMG

This part of the analysis is based on a study of those FMGs who achieved immigrant status in the United States during the period 1961-1971, [32] and focuses on the characteristics of that cohort in terms of: (1) the method whereby, and the time elapsing before, they achieved immigrant status; (2) the experiences of the cohort with respect to the ECFMG examination, licensure, and areas and modes of practice; and (3) the employment status of the unlicensed physicians in the cohort.

As previously indicated, foreign physicians have been allowed to enter the United States in one of two ways: (1) directly as immigrants, with no constraints on the length of time they are allowed to remain; or (2) as nonimmigrants, increasingly in the form of exchange visitors seeking further training and having the option of adjusting to immigrant status while in the United States. Of a cohort of foreign physicians achieving immigrant status during the period 1961-1971, the proportion doing so by adjusting status increased each year, from over 12 percent during the years 1961-1965 to nearly double that proportion in 1968-1969 and nearly four times (47 percent) that proportion in 1970-1971 (table 2-11). The unusually high rate in the last period can be attributed to a relaxation in 1970 of the law requiring exchange visitors to leave the United States for two years before seeking immigrant status. Two-thirds of those adjusting status had originally entered the United States as exchange visitors.

For those adjusting status, the average time elapsing between the year they entered the United States as nonimmigrants and the year they became immigrants was over four years; about 17 percent managed to change in less than two years, and about 13 percent waited eight years or more (table 2-12). The surprisingly large proportion of those in the last group may be explained by the fact that, before the relaxation of this requirement, many physicians who had entered the United States as exchange visitors left for two years as required by the law and again entered the United States as exchange visitors. For some, the year of entry recorded was that of second entry; for others, it was the year of first entry, which would put a number of them into the group recorded as waiting eight years or more.

Table 2-11
Method of Admission for a Cohort of Physicians Admitted to the United States as Immigrants during Specified Years

Year of Admission	*Percentage Adjusting Status (1)*	*Percentage Using Occupational Preference (2)*[a]	*Total Number (3)*
1961-1965	13	0	9,244
1966-1967	24	31	6,409
1968-1969	24	32	5,817
1970-1971	47	25	7,102
Total	26	29[b]	28,572

Source: J.C. Kleinman, R.J. Weiss, and D.S. Felsenthal, "Immigrant Physicians. Results of a Cohort Study," *Inquiry* 12(1975):193-203.

[a]Consists of those members of occupational groups declared by the U.S. Department of Labor as being in short supply.

[b]The denominator used to calculate the total proportion for that group was the 19,328 physicians shown in column 3, as being admitted during the period 1966-1971.

Table 2-12
Foreign Physicians Admitted to the United States as Immigrants through Adjustment of Status during the Period 1961-1971[a]

	Year of Admission				
Number of Years before Admission	*1961-65 (%)*	*1966-67 (%)*	*1968-69 (%)*	*1970-71 (%)*	*Total (%)*
0-1	27	17	17	13	17
2-3	20	29	29	27	27
4-5	23	18	20	30	24
6-7	17	15	22	21	19
8+	13	21	12	9	13
Total	100	100	100	100	100
Number	1,165	1,534	1,395	3,363	7,457

Source: J.C. Kleinman, R.J. Weiss, and D.S. Felsenthal, "Immigrant Physicians. Results of a Cohort Study," *Inquiry* 12(1975):193-203.

[a]Percentage distribution by number of years between original entry and year of admission.

Of the total cohort, 88 percent took the ECFMG examination for the first time before achieving immigrant status, but only 70 percent passed. The proportion of those passing, however, varied from one segment of the cohort to another: Of the group achieving immigrant status during the period 1961–1967, about 70 percent had passed, with the proportion declining to 60 percent for the 1968–1969 group and rising to 75 percent for the 1970–1971 group. These figures apply, of course, only to those foreign physicians registered with the ECFMG. It is estimated that, if the "underground" physicians were taken into account, 49 percent of the immigrants could be considered as not having passed the examination prior to admission—in other words, only 51 percent instead of 70 percent in all had passed prior to admission.

With regard to those of the whole cohort whose records were in the ECFMG file and for whom the relevant years were known, the following pattern emerged with respect to their passing of the ECFMG examination, in relation to the year in which they were admitted to the United States as immigrants:

Twenty-seven percent had passed more than four years before admission.

Ten percent had passed three to four years before admission.

Twenty percent had passed one to two years before admission.

Twelve percent had passed in the same year as admission.

Ten percent had passed one to two years after admission.

Three percent had passed three to four years after admission.

One percent had passed more than four years after admission.

Seventeen percent had not passed.

Regarding those physicians admitted as direct immigrants in the occupational-preference category (about one-third of the total), the failure rate was higher than that for those adjusting status, 27 percent as opposed to 17 percent for the years 1968–1971.

Of all who passed the ECFMG examination, 54 percent had passed after one attempt, 74 percent after two attempts, 94 percent after three attempts, and the remainder after four or more attempts.

The primary indicator of acceptance in the health-care system of the United States is licensure. Regarding the immigrant cohort studied, licensure data were perforce limited to that portion of the cohort that could be matched to the AMA file—7,270 individuals or about one-fourth of the cohort. The life table that follows shows the cumulative rate of licensure for a hypothetical cohort of immigrant physicians, based on the experience of the actual cohort studied:

Period Ending:	*Cumulative Percentage Licensed*
Before admission	5
Same year as admission	13
1 year after admission	34
2 years after	47
3 years after	59
4 years after	68
5 years after	75
6 years after	84
7 years after	89
8 years after	90
9 years after	92
10 years after	93

From these figures, it can be seen that by the end of the third year after admission, over half the immigrants were licensed; by the end of the fifth year, three-quarters were licensed; but by the end of the tenth year, 7 percent were still unlicensed—the latter not including the unlicensed "underground." Another study cited by the author of the same report found that 42 percent of USMGs had been licensed by the end of the first year after graduation, 55 percent by the end of the third year, 70 percent by the end of the fifth year, and 91 percent by the end of the eighth year. Thus, except for the first year concerned, the differences in licensure rates between immigrant FMGs and USMGs were small.

This information is pertinent to those of the 7,270 immigrant physicians who were fully licensed. About 40 percent were not fully licensed, among whom 5 percent were interns, 19 percent were residents, and 15 percent were not in training.

Within the cohort as a whole, 3,792 individuals were identified as not being in training but undertaking direct patient care as a major activity. Of these, 17 percent were unlicensed. Table 2–13 compares these unlicensed physicians with those who were licensed, in terms of type and place of practice. The unlicensed group shows larger proportions in nongovernmental and state hospitals and smaller proportions in private practice. Also, among the unlicensed the proportion unclassified according to type of employment is much larger than among the licensed.

Examination of the time interval elapsing between the end of the first internship and the year of achievement of immigrant status revealed two important points: (1) 37 percent of the immigrants had no internship listed (that is, they had gone directly into either residency or another type of employment); and (2) of those who were either serving their internship at the time or had completed it, 51 percent completed it before their admission as immigrants. The proportion varied over time, from 43 percent for those admitted during the period 1961–1965, to 61 percent for those admitted in 1970–1971.

In the case of residency training, only 22 percent of the cohort had no residency listed. Of those who had, 32 percent had completed it before their admission as immigrants. With regard to specialty-board certification, the proportion obtaining such certification declined, from 31 percent for those admitted during the period 1961–1965, to 19 percent for those admitted in 1966–1967, and to 11 percent each for those admitted in 1968–1969 and 1970–1971. For those immigrant physicians matched to the AMA file, table 2-8 shows their pattern of distribution with regard to specialty.

The Noncertified FMG

Although the literature has disclosed a great deal about the utilization of FMGs in the health system of the United States, little has been published on the experience of FMGs prior to entering the United States. One study, however, attempted to shed some light on that subject. [31] The population studied was the total cohort of candidates taking the ECFMG examination on 24 January 1973, in the United States. By definition, the candidates were not certified by the ECFMG and thus were also not licensed to practice medicine in the United States, although, as previously indicated, many unlicensed FMGs are not only working in the health system but are providing direct patient care.

Among the candidates studied, 57 percent of the 850 respondents claimed to have had specialty training prior to coming to the United States. Of those having such training, 59 percent had been certified in a specialty, the most common specialties being obstetrics and gynecology, surgery, pediatrics, internal medicine, and anesthesiology. The tendency to focus on these areas of specialization, prior to entry to the United States, could be a reflection of one or both of the following factors: (1) awareness that particular specialties in the United States were short of necessary manpower induced candidates to prepare themselves in those fields in order to ensure their employment in the United States if they were to decide to go there; and (2) interest in those particular areas of practice that were, coincidentally, experiencing manpower shortages in the United States. In either case, FMGs on the whole in the United States have inclined strongly toward these areas of practice.

In addition, 81 percent of the respondents claimed they had worked as

Table 2-13
Type of Employment, by Licensure Status, of a Cohort of Immigrant Physicians in the United States Who Were Not in Training Programs but Whose Major Activity Was Patient Care, 1971

Type of Employment	*Licensed (%)*	*Unlicensed (%)*	*Total (%)*
Solo practice	29	11	26
Other private practice	23	11	22
Medical school	5	7	6
Nongovernment hospital	17	40	20
City or county hospital	7	6	6
State hospital	9	15	10
Veterans hospital	6	3	5
Other federal hospital	1	4	2
Nonhospital employment	3	3	3
Total	100	100	100
Number: total	2,990	481	3,471
employment status unknown	175	146	321

Source: J.C. Kleinman, R.J. Weiss, and D.S. Felsenthal, "Immigrant Physicians. Results of a Cohort Study," *Inquiry* 12(1975):193-203.

Note: Only those immigrant physicians matched to the AMA file are included in this table.

physicians prior to entering the United States. Of those with such experience, 63 percent had had specialty training; of those without such experience, only 32 percent had had specialty training.

Table 2-14 shows the proportions, by country of medical education, of those candidates with specialty training and those with work experience prior to entering the United States. Mexico shows the lowest proportions in both cases, while Cuba ranks among those with the highest proportions. European countries in general show relatively low proportions in both cases, compared with countries of South America and the Middle East.

The past experience of the respondents was compared with their employment status at the time of taking the ECFMG examination. The proportions with training or experience were significantly higher among those employed in the health field than among those not so employed.

Table 2-14
Non-ECFMG-Certified Physicians: Their Specialty Training and Work Experience Prior to Entering the United States, by Area of Medical Education, 1973

Area of Medical Education	*Number of Respondents*	*Percentage with Speicalty Training*	*Percentage with Work Experience*
Cuba	56	73	72
Mexico	31	47	48
Philippines	285	55	85
India, Pakistan, and Sri Lanka	160	49	77
Middle East	16	63	78
Far East	63	56	80
Central America	23	58	91
South America	59	69	76
Europe	138	56	72
Other	19	66	68
Total	850	57	81

Source: J.C. Kleinman, U.C. Brandt, and R.J. Weiss, "Postgraduate Training and Work Experience of Non-ECFMG Certified Physicians in the U.S.," *Medical Care* 13(1975): 205-208.

Note: Data refer to a sample of candidates taking the ECFMG examination on 24 January 1973 in the United States. The proportions were adjusted for year of graduation since some countries, such as Cuba, were represented primarily by older graduates and others, such as Mexico, by more recent graduates.

Despite the fact that so large a portion of the sample had postgraduate clinical experience, only 21 percent passed the ECFMG examination and 83 percent had taken the examination at least once before. Even more noteworthy is the fact that 60 percent of the respondents were employed in the health field, and 44 percent had patient-care responsibilities.

3 Forces Conditioning Physician Migration

The excessive migration of physicians is conditioned by a multiplicity of forces operating at various levels. At the international level it is symptomatic of political, economic, and social imbalances in the world system. At the national level it is symptomatic of imbalances in the demand/supply market for physicians, with the imbalance favoring the demand aspect in the recipient country and the supply aspect in the donor country. Imbalances at the national level find their roots in the overall asymmetrical relations between nations at opposite ends of the development scale.

Physicians generally migrate *from* countries where the effective economic demand for them is less than the supply. They generally migrate *to* countries where the opposite is true. In exceptional cases, they migrate from countries because of political factors largely unrelated to the physician demand/supply market.

The forces that condition the demand/supply market vary from country to country. In the United States, the preponderance of demand is primarily the result of: (1) the overall rising affluence of the country reflected in a rising level of disposable personal income, a broad coverage of the population by health-insurance schemes, and expanding government subsidies to the health sector; (2) the population's increasing knowledge about health and the availability of health technology, and its increasing awareness of its right to health care—both of these resulting from rising levels of education; and (3) changes in the age distribution of the population that resulted in a growing number of elderly persons, who, as a whole, require more medical services over longer periods of time than do younger persons. On the other hand, the shortage of physician supply in the United States has been caused largely by the medical profession's desire, in the name of quality, to restrict its numbers—through the system of accreditation it established with respect to academic and training institutions, through its allowing to enter the profession only those who had been graduated from an accredited professional school, and through its establishment of a barrage of licensure requirements. The generous contributions of the government to health research did much to raise the levels of medical technology with respect to the more esoteric diseases, but this took place at the expense of care to broader segments of society.

In the countries that are primarily donors, imbalances in the demand/

supply market are largely caused by unequal distribution of wealth within the country concerned; that is, large segments of the population have so little personal income that they can ill afford the services of costly health manpower. Moreover, government expenditure on health is usually very low both in absolute terms and in relation to total government expenditure. On the other hand, the donor country tends to produce more physicians than it can sustain, in terms of the medical services its people can afford to purchase. To this can be added the fact that the physician's education may be largely irrelevant to the most pervasive needs of the masses, that is, their need for primary health care as opposed to sophisticated and costly medical care in hospitals. The factors underlying the overproduction of physicians in relation to the effective economic demand for medical services, as well as those underlying the manner in which physicians in the donor country are trained, form a large part of the story of why a country becomes a donor of physicians.

International Forces

Through the WHO Multinational Study of the International Migration of Physicians and Nurses, which may be considered the parent of the case study presented in this book, it was possible to gain a broad understanding of the international forces that induce the migration of health manpower. The large number of physicians migrating to the United States illustrates, perhaps more sharply than do other patterns of physician migration, the interplay of forces at the international level. In this regard, therefore, it may be worthwhile to recapitulate certain findings and conclusions emanating from the multinational study before going into greater detail about those forces specific only to the United States as the primary recipient of migrant physicians and those specific to individual large-scale donors of physicians to the United States.

Evidence suggests that the excessive migration of physicians, like that of other manpower, whether highly educated or not, is largely conditioned by, and therefore symptomatic of, political, economic, and social imbalances in the world system. The recognition of these factors does not, however, obscure the fact that the world consists of countries at varying levels of development and affluence, and that the flow of health manpower has been not only from the poorest to the richest countries but also from poorer to somewhat richer countries and, if one takes into account health manpower in technical-assistance programs, from richer to poorer countries.

Nevertheless, the predominant flows of health manpower have been toward the wealthiest and most industrially developed market-economy countries, reflecting an international political and economic order in which the weaker economies have been subordinated to the priorities of the stronger ones. In this context, migration can be described as a flow process analogous to that of other physical matter, for example, the flow of water through a pipe. The flow, in either case, results from a *driving force* at the source of the flow and a *pulling force* at the other end. These forces arise because a characteristic quantity has different magnitudes in the two areas between which there is a flow. Without the driving force at the source of the flow, however, and regardless of the pulling force at the other end, there would be little if any flow. The volume of the flow in response to a given driving force can, theoretically, be controlled by valves at either end of the flow channel. In practice, however, very few countries have been both willing and able to develop an effective system of controls against whatever driving forces may exist; while even fewer countries, if any, have succeeded in creating an internal situation in which driving forces do not exist and in which controlling forces are therefore unnecessary. It follows, then, that the magnitude of the flow is largely determined by the way in which the control mechanisms at the receiving end of the potential flow channel are manipulated. This has been clearly shown by observed fluctuations in the migration patterns of manpower, generally to the more affluent countries of the world. Such fluctuations have represented responses to the changing laws of those countries concerning the admission of foreigners; the changing laws, in turn, reflect changes in the manpower-supply/demand market.

That this theory holds with respect to the migration of physicians was shown in the WHO multinational study. With regard to the United States, earlier chapters of this book have already shown the effect that changes in U.S. laws had on the volume and sources of the inflow of foreign physicians and, in turn, on certain of their characteristics as a group. Undoubtedly, the most recent legislation enacted in the United States (described in appendix A) will just as effectively alter the inflow of physicians.

While the volume of migration into a particular country can be regulated by that country, this does not necessarily (and certainly not automatically or immediately) alter the driving forces in the donor country, which stem largely from inequalities at the international level. It is clear, therefore, that ultimately only reducing the gross inequalities between nations will remove the root determinants of large-scale migration.

In this context it is important to note the *extent* of inequality at the international level. In 1972 the industrialized market-economy countries, with only 17 percent of the world's population, accounted for two-thirds of the world's output of goods and services; they control an even larger share of the world's manufacturing, research, and scientific capability. At the other extreme, 26 percent of the world's population lived in countries where the average annual income per capita was less than $200, and where total output was less than 3 percent of global output. If China were included in the calculation, it would mean that nearly half the world's population received less than 7 percent of the world's income. [30]

While in 1972 the per-capita gross national product (GNP) in the developing world was just over U.S. $300, in a number of countries, such as India, Pakistan, Bangladesh, and Sri Lanka, it was less than half that amount. All these countries are heavy donors of health manpower. The degree of poverty in these countries can be better gauged if one considers that per-capita GNP in the United States at that time was U.S. $6,200. [29]

The gross imbalance at the international level is matched by a similar phenomenon at the national level. In most developing countries, the richest 10 percent of households typically receive about 40 percent of personal income, the poorest 40 percent receive 15 percent or less, and the very poorest 20 percent receive about 5 percent. [30] In several respects this inequality *within* countries appears to derive from the extensive inequality *between* countries. In the broad areas of international interaction—trade, technology transfer, private investment, monetary arrangements, military activities, and aid—as well as in the way the international system of negotiation and agreement operates, the constraints are such that the poor in a country have little if any opportunity to share in whatever benefit might accrue to the country through international transactions.

With regard to the migration of physicians, this implies that the purchasing power of large segments of the population is so low that they cannot afford, either directly or through social-insurance schemes, the services of physicians, whose education—and, therefore, utilization—are costly. The result of this is the unemployment or underemployment of a proportion of physicians, many of whom are obliged to migrate if they wish to use the skills in which they have invested.

Since the end of World War II, the increasing affluence in some of the highly industrialized countries of the West has led to rapidly increasing demands for services of all sorts, including those for personal health care. The increasing cost of such care (caused, among other things, by the use of highly sophisticated technology; the installation of luxurious, comfort-giving, but relatively nonessential equipment; and the considerable funds poured into research) was largely at the expense of domestic health-manpower production. The resultant gross imbalance between the demand for personal health care and the supply of health manpower had to be rapidly rectified. The response was a wide opening of the door to health manpower from abroad. The fact that such manpower may have been obtained at virtually no cost to the importing countries forms a part of the story of the asymmetric relationships between nations.

The period since World War II was also one of political liberation in the third world: Over eighty new nations emerged, and over a billion people were liberated from colonialism. But political independence did not automatically liberate such nations from their economic dependence on rich countries, a dependence rooted in the international system of institutions created largely by the industrialized countries, essentially for the purpose of enhancing and protecting the affluence and the life styles to which their societies had become accustomed and to which the third world had perforce made a significant contribution. The question of who was dependent on whom during the period of colonization has not been fully answered. However, the liberated nations, left with limited financial resources, a dearth of trained national manpower, an inadequate infrastructure, and limited opportunities to use internally the raw materials they had, were far from achieving the economic independence needed to complete and secure their political independence.

While there are signs that the third world is gaining momentum in its search for collective economic security, large segments of that world continue to live in abject poverty. To lay the blame for this continuing situation *entirely* on the affluent market-economy countries would be unfair, given that political autonomy does allow power holders in even poor countries considerable room for maneuverability with respect to the choice of a feasible path toward national development. The People's Republic of China, one of the poorest and most populous countries of the world, appears to have effectively demonstrated this.

Although the governing elites in virtually all third-world countries have generally proclaimed themselves in favor of raising the living standards of the poor masses, their strategies for development have tended to favor the privileged few. Many conceived the objectives of development in terms of Western living standards and assumed, as did the entire United Nations system during the so-called First Development Decade, that widespread poverty and employment problems in the developing world would be *rapidly* overcome by measures taken to accelerate overall economic growth, regardless of the path pursued to that end. While GNP per capita grew exceptionally fast during the 1960s in most developing countries, it tended to to be concentrated in relatively limited parts of their economies, mostly in those sectors using capital-intensive techniques and having few links with the traditional rural sectors or the informal urban sectors, which between them account for by far the greater part of the employment potential in most developing countries. Relatively little attention was paid to the health and welfare of this potentially productive population, or to the development of education and training programs aimed at making that population productive. As a result, the benefits of growth, and in particular opportunities for productive employment, went mainly to a very small segment of the total population.

The pattern of income and wealth distribution within a country both reflects and determines the pattern of consumption of goods and services, including those related to health. In many developing countries the pattern related to health imitated that of the industrialized market-economy countries. This is evident in the types of health manpower produced, in the manner in which they are educated and trained, in where and how they are employed, and in the types and quantities of nonlabor resources provided (for example, buildings, equipment, money) and the way these are distributed. That the health problems in developing countries were essentially different from those in the more affluent countries was not taken into account, although the eagerly sought (and just as eagerly provided) support and guidance from foreign agencies should not be ignored. The nature of the evolution of the health professions and services in most parts of the developing world, and the role of foreign agencies in that evolution, appear to have been largely conditioned by two elements, one social and the other structural.

The *social* element is the fact that the members of the power-holding elite in the countries concerned largely share the values and tastes of affluent societies, and are thus willing partners in the perpetuation of the patterns of production and consumption obtaining in those societies. This elite includes not only the economic elite (those who are in the upper income brackets and/or control the distribution of income and wealth), but also the health elite (part of which belongs to the economic elite), including decision makers in the health sector, health planners, health administrators, and certain categories of professional health personnel, such as physicians, dentists, and health researchers. The decisions made by these groups (on policies, technology, administration, and resources) are based on the needs of that layer of society to which these groups are exposed, and whose lifestyles induce a pattern of illness that is not representative of the country as a whole but which resembles that of affluent societies everywhere. The pattern of disease of the elite would thus receive priority in the country's health services and teaching institutions. The fact that most students and teachers, especially those in medicine, are recruited from this segment of the population compounds the problem. Furthermore, to a large extent this segment of the population also owns and/or controls the institutions that produce health manpower and those that deliver health services.

The *structural* element conditioning the evolution of the health professions and services is the competitive advantage that foreign agencies have in marketing their technology, and the vigor with which they promote the acceptance of such technology in the developing world. Almost no country can resist the temptation of an expensive and sophisticated teaching hospital, whose facilities are designed for the treatment of rare diseases and the provision of exquisite personal care for a few, and whose teaching and learning are oriented toward health care in conditions of comfort and luxury that the vast majority of people cannot afford. Moreover, few health workers, once exposed to the glamour of such technology, desire to work in less glamorous settings or to deal with the ordinary diseases afflicting the masses.

Imported technology can hardly avoid reflecting the values and tastes of the exporting country. To the extent that this is so, the technology becomes less relevant to the highest-priority health needs of people in the importing country. Health manpower trained by means of, and for the further use of, such technology become largely irrelevant themselves. Where more of such manpower is produced than can be used, the excess will migrate to where their skills can be afforded and their professional and economic expectations met. More often than not, the exporter of the technology thus becomes the recipient of health manpower suited to its own requirements.

While the poor stand to gain little from much of the technology transferred, there are others who do benefit: the providers of the technology, including the multinational corporations that either sell directly to the countries concerned or maintain within them subsidiary firms that produce commodities for internal consumption, and possibly for export; the academics and research workers in the affluent countries, who use the developing world as a happy hunting ground for credits in teaching and research (many of the subjects taught and studies conducted are of little relevance to the highest-priority health problems in the developing world); the academics and researchers in the developing world, who receive research grants, fellowships, and subsidized travel abroad for study and for meetings of experts (which, again, are not particularly relevant to the problems of the developing world); the medical practitioners, who are both a product of and a vehicle for the use of such technology, and who seek concrete compensation for the time and effort they have invested in specialized training; and the small segment of the population that can afford health care involving sophisticated technology.

In terms of programs, personnel, institutions, and structures, those responsible for the health systems of their countries have several options. In many cases, however, the "edifice complex" has prevailed, resulting in the construction of prestigious teaching hospitals for the purpose of producing health manpower to meet some obscure, ill-defined, but allegedly "high and international" standards of excellence. Throughout much of the developing world, national health administrations have aspired to such standards of excellence, if only in order that their medical schools may achieve "international recognition," that is, recognition by the affluent countries of the West. Such recognition generally implies merely that the products of such schools possess qualifications that are negotiable in the international market for skills. Few of those possessing such qualifications can resist the temptation of testing their worth in that market. For thousands, the first step toward that end has been taking the ECFMG examination.

It is evident that migration does not occur in a vacuum but is conditioned by a combination of forces working at both ends of the migratory channel. These forces include driving forces at the source of the flow (forces that determine essentially whether or not there will be an outflow) and pulling forces at the destination of the flow. Pulling forces vary in strength from country to country; the countries with the strongest pulling forces determine the direction of the flow. The flow of physicians to the United States has been far greater than that to any other country of the world (about half of all migrant physicians in the world are in the United States) because of that country's exceptionally powerful pulling forces. While these forces may have little to do with the flora and fauna of the country, the hospitable nature of its people, or other such attributes (that are equally applicable to other countries, including the donor countries), they have much to do with the supply/demand market for physicians in the United States and the political forces conditioning that market.

Forces in the United States

The large inflow of foreign physicians to the United States has occurred basically because the local production of physicians had failed to keep pace with the demand for medical services. In this section of the chapter an attempt is made to describe the factors conditioning the demand for medical services, those conditioning the supply of physicians, the imbalances in the demand/supply market, and the ways in which the nation has tried to redress the imbalances.

Factors Conditioning Demand

During the past three decades, consumers and government agencies in the United States have diverted increasing amounts of their annual budgets toward the purchase of health-care services. Some of the factors contributing to the rising demand for health services are population growth, and changes in the age distribution of a population, increased education and sophistication regarding health, and the ability of the medical profession to provide more and better services. More important, however, are factors that have enabled buyers to translate their desires into demand; such factors include increased disposable personal income, widespread health-insurance coverage, and expanding government subsidies.

Of all the factors conditioning the demand for health services, particularly medical services, in the United States, the rising affluence of the population was the primary factor in either facilitating the emergence or shaping the nature of other important factors.

The GNP of the United States grew by 353 percent between the years 1950 and 1973. While much of this increase was attributable to rising prices, even in constant 1958 dollars the GNP increased by 92 percent in that period. Because the growth of the GNP was more rapid than population growth, per-capita disposable income increased from $1,364 in 1950 to $4,195 in 1973, an increase of 208 percent or, in constant 1958 dollars, 76 percent. With the rise in per-capita income, the proportion of persons considered to be living below the poverty line was nearly halved, decreasing from about 22 percent in 1959 to about 13 percent in 1972. [60]

Although affluence in the form of better nutrition, housing, and sanitary facilities alleviated some of the problems associated with poverty, affluence also translated into an excessive consumption of rich foods, alcohol, and cigarettes; too little physical exercise; too much stress resulting from the drive toward greater affluence, and so on—all of which created new health hazards. Because money to pay for health care was available, greater demands were addressed to the health-care system—demands not only for more health services, but also for better and more personal care for a greater number of people.

Affluence, combined with revolutionary advances in medical technology (which were largely stimulated by affluence), helped change the characteristics of the population considerably. For example, the rate of population growth had decreased from 18 percent during the period 1950–1960 to 13 percent during the subsequent decade, [60] mainly as a result of a lower fertility rate that was due in part to technological advances in contraceptive methods. One might have expected the slower rate of population growth to have led to either a steady or a declining rate of demand for health services. This did not happen, however, because the population was also growing older—partly because fewer babies were being born, and partly because access to better care in their earlier years had allowed more people to live to an advanced age. In 1973 over 10 percent of the total population was over 65 years old, compared with only half that proportion in 1930. [60] On a per-capita basis, older people suffer from more disabilities and chronic illnesses than do younger people, and therefore require more medical services at all stages of care: Physician visits per person per year increase considerably with age; hospital-admission rates are higher for older people; when hospitalized, older people tend to require longer hospital stays; and after discharge from the hospital, older people are likely to require longer periods of time for rehabilitation and more continuing medical care, either at home, in a nursing home, or in an extended-care facility.

The population of the United States has also become better educated; 60 percent of those over the age of 25 years have completed secondary education. The number of bachelor-of-arts degrees awarded annually rose by 373 percent between 1940 and 1971, while the number of doctoral degrees rose by 970 percent. [60] People's increasing level of education made them more knowledgeable about medical care and more aware and demanding of their right to care. Growth in the number of educated people, combined with affluence, led to a growing concern about equality of opportunity, with access to health care being increasingly regarded as a right of all rather than as a privilege of the more prosperous. This concern led to greatly increasing government support for programs aimed at making it easier for the aged and the poor to obtain health care, for example, health insurance for the medically indigent (Medicaid) and for the aged (Medicare). These facilitating mechanisms, in turn, led to even greater demands for health care.

Health-insurance coverage has grown at a phenomenal rate over the last three decades. Whereas in 1940 only 12 million people were insured for hospital expenses, 5 million for surgical expenses, and 3 million for regular medical expenses, by 1973 the numbers climbed to 182, 169, and 152 million, respectively. Thus, while less than 10 percent of the resident population in 1940 was insured for hospital expenses, 85 percent of the population in 1973 was so insured. The proportion covered for surgical expenses rose from 4 to 79 percent in that period. As for coverage for medical expenses other than surgery, the proportion rose from 2 to 71 percent, but this coverage was mostly for care related to a hospital stay; in 1973 only 34 percent of the population had insurance for medical care outside the hospital (table 3-1 and figure 3-1).

That portion of the consumer's *hospital* expenses covered either by private insurance or by the government grew over the years, until by 1974 the consumer's out-of-pocket payment for hospital care amounted, on the average, to only about 10 percent of the total: Private insurance paid 36 percent, and the government (through Medicare or Medicaid) paid 53 percent. With regard to physicians' fees, however, the consumer's out-of-pocket payment amounted to 39 percent of the total, or four times the proportion payable for hospital expenses. Thus, in 1974 the per-capita out-of-pocket expenditure was $34.37 for physicians' services but only $19.90 for hospital care. [60]

The fact that the consumer paid a far smaller share of hospital expenses than of physicians' fees is undoubtedly a strong reason why the demand for hospital care grew much more rapidly than that for physicians' services—even though from the national viewpoint hospital care was more than twice as expensive as any other care ($190 per capita in 1974, as opposed to $88 for physicians' services). Admissions to all hospitals in the

Table 3-1
Proportion of People in the United States with Health-Insurance Protection, by Type of Coverage, Selected Years, 1940-1973

		Percentage of Population Covered for:		
End of Year	*Population (Thousands) (1)*	*Hospital Expenses (2)*	*Surgical Expenses (3)*	*Regular Medical Expenses (4)*
1940	131,970	9	4	2
1945	139,586	23	9	3
1950	156,472	49	35	14
1955	170,499	62	52	32
1960	185,370	70	63	47
1965	199,278	75	69	58
1970	209,539	82	77	69
1971	211,578	83	77	69
1972	213,046	84	77	69
1973	214,583	85	79	71

Sources (column 1): United States Department of Health, Education, and Welfare, Public Health Service, Health Resources Administration, National Center for Health Statistics, *Health Resources Statistics Reported from the National Center for Health Statistics 1975* (Rockville, Md.: U.S. Department of Health, Education, and Welfare, 1976); (column 2, 3, and 4): idem, Bureau of Health Planning and Resources Development, *Trends Affecting U.S. Health Care System,* DHEW Publication no. (HRA) 76,14503 (Rockville, Md.: U.S. Department of Health, Education, and Welfare, 1976).

United States totaled about 34.4 million in 1973, or 86 percent more than in 1950. This rise was more than double the 38 percent increase in population between 1950 and 1973. [60] In other words, a large proportion of the rise in hospital admissions was probably due to the fact that hospital care was less costly to the individual than were physicians' services. The demand for medical services in hospitals rose to the point where the domestic supply of physicians was insufficient to meet that demand. The story of the foreign medical graduate in the United States thus became part of the larger story of how the government tried to resolve the imbalance between demand and supply in the country's health sector, and particularly with respect to hospital services.

Factors Conditioning Supply

The supply of physicians in the United States is conditioned essentially by the following factors:

1. how medicine as a profession developed over the years and established early control over the most important avenues of entry to the profession: through the system of accreditation it established with respect to academic and training institutions, through its allowing only those to enter the profession who were graduates of an accredited professional school, and through its establishment of licensure requirements;
2. how the profession succeeded in prescribing its own styles and standards of work, and thereby in maximizing its freedom and its economic returns;
3. how the AMA emerged as the spokesman for organized medicine, and thus as a powerful political force in the nation;
4. how, with the backing of the AMA and the government's funding of health research, technological specialization, together with its elaborate and expensive facilities and equipment and its array of specialists, superspecialists, and nonspecialists, was grafted onto a profession of generalists engaged in solo, private, office-based, and fee-for-service practice.

The following discussion attempts to portray, along these lines, the manner in which the "shortage" of physicians or, as recent thinking has it, the "maldistribution" of physicians in the United States developed.

Reform of Medical Education. The strength of the medical profession in the United States has long rested on its success in restricting its own numbers. The first successful large-scale effort to restrict the supply of physicians dates back to the early years of the present century, when both medical schools and physicians were plentiful (although of dubious quality in many instances, according to reports at the time). It has been estimated that between 1800 and 1900 over 400 medical schools were founded. However, for various reasons many of them failed, so that by 1900 there were only 160, most of them small, profit-making trade schools with rather facile requirements for both admission and graduation. Subsequent events effected a 50 percent reduction in this smaller number.

The early effort to restrict the number of medical schools and, at the same time, to limit the supply but improve the quality of graduates was stimulated by an inordinately frank report prepared by the educator Abraham Flexner and published by the Carnegie Foundation in 1910. [23] The report, based on an investigation of every medical school existing at the time, exposed for the first time the conditions prevailing in each school, by name. Some twenty schools investigated are reported to have closed even before the report was prepared, in order to avoid the devastating critique that might otherwise have been their lot. Others were more courageous, but few were spared. Assessments such as "appalling," "miserable," and

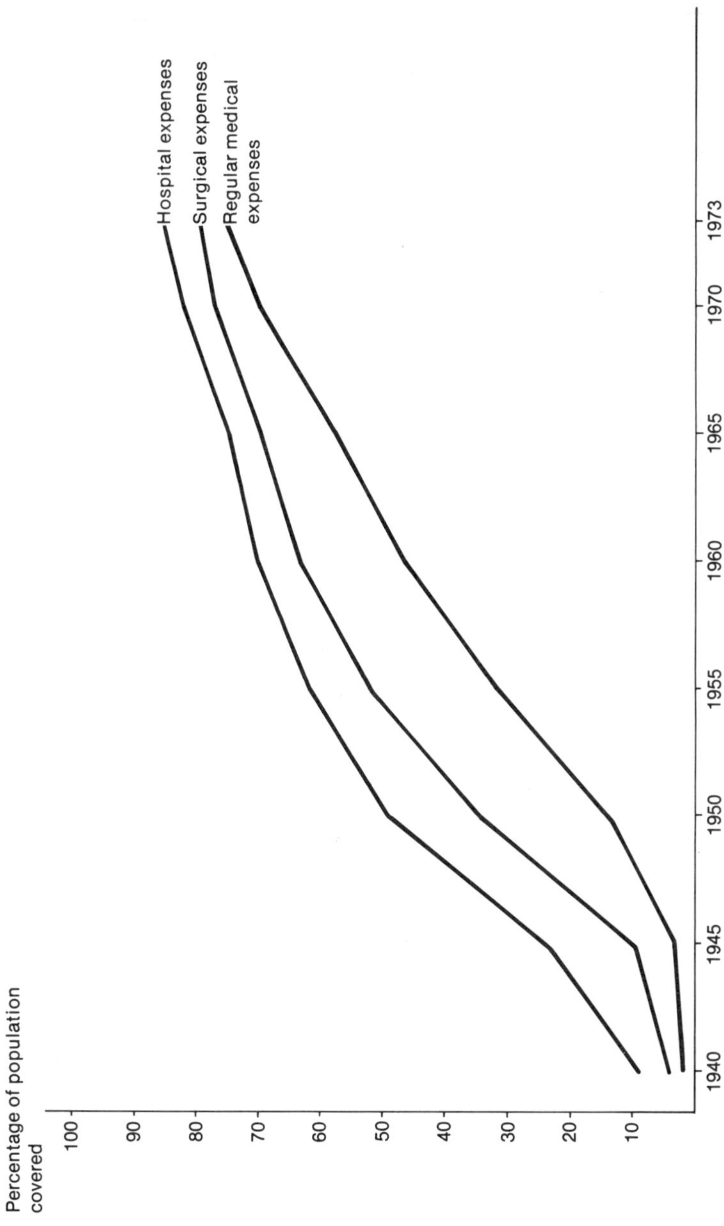

Source: Table 3–1

Figure 3–1. Proportion of People in the United States with Health-Insurance Protection, by Type of Coverage, Selected Years, 1940–1973.

"utterly wretched" appeared profusely in the pages of the report. Only three schools escaped censure on all counts: Harvard, Johns Hopkins, and Western Reserve.

Using Johns Hopkins as the model for medical education, the Flexner report strongly urged the provision of full-time teaching staff and the access of students and staff to laboratory and hospital facilities, so that teaching and research could be combined in each school. The report also strongly endorsed the notion that medical education was a function of universities, thereby denying any role for proprietary schools, which at the time greatly outnumbered university-based schools. Moreover, it emphasized the need for more stringent admission requirements and higher standards of teaching.

What may have been most surprising, even to the most ardent reformists, was the report's recommendation that the number of medical schools be reduced to 31, each giving a four-year course and producing no more than 70 graduates per year, that is, a total of no more than 2,170 graduates per year. That the report, or even the prospect of the report, had the intended impact is evident from table 3-2, which shows that by 1920 there were only 85 schools, as compared with 162 in 1906 (the year before the investigation started) and 131 in 1910 (the year the report was published). Annual production also decreased, from over 5,000 in 1906 to about 3,000 in 1920. During the same period, the number of physicians per 10,000 population dropped from 16 to 13, remaining at the latter level through the years of the economic depression and rising only slightly through the 1950s. [58] Moreover, whereas in 1905 only 5 schools required any college preparation for admission, ten years later 85 schools prescribed a minimum of one or two years of such preparation. By 1932, every recognized medical school and most of the state licensing boards required at least two years, many required three, and several required a college degree. With the rising standards of entry to medical school, state licensing requirements also rose: by 1925, forty-nine boards required that candidates for their examinations be graduates of a medical college, and forty-six states refused to recognize graduates of low-grade medical schools as qualifying for licensure. Since the AMA Council on Medical Education was the only body assessing the quality of the nation's medical schools, the AMA and thus the medical profession effectively gained control over the regulation of medical education. [45]

Although on the one hand the success of the reforms in undergraduate medical education could be seen in terms of the rising prestige and economic status of the physician, the excellence of the nation's medical schools, and the AMA's unification of the institutions of medicine, the reforms also gave rise to or aggravated other problems. One serious, long-term, and negative social effect of the drive toward the standardization of medical education

Table 3-2
Physicians, Medical Schools, Students, and Graduates in the United States, Selected Years, 1810-1957

	Physicians		*Medical Schools*		
Year	*Number*	*Number per 10,000 Population*	*Number*	*Students (Number)*	*Graduates (Number)*
1810			5		
1850			52		
1870	60,000	15.0	75		
1880	82,000	16.3	100	11,826	3,241
1900	119,749	15.7	160	25,171	5,214
1906	134,688	15.8	162	25,204	5,364
1910	135,000	14.6	131	21,526	4,440
1918	147,812	14.1	90	13,630	2,670
1923	145,966	13.0	80	16,960	3,120
1929	152,503	12.5	76	20,878	4,446
1934	161,359	12.8	77	22,799	5,035
1940	175,163	13.3	77	21,271	5,097
1949	201,277	13.5	78	23,670	5,094
1957	226,625	13.2	85	29,130	6,796

Source: United States Department of Health, Education, and Welfare, *Health Manpower Source Book,* Public Health Service Publication no. 263, section 9 (Washington, D.C.: U.S. Government Printing Office, 1959).

Note: Data for some years may not accord with those cited elsewhere, owing to differences in coverage.

was the closing of schools for black students. Of eight such schools existing before the advent of the Flexner report, four closed before 1914, a fifth in 1915, and a sixth in 1923. During their short existence, these six schools, most of them founded after 1880, had produced a thousand physicians, about half of whom had passed state board examinations. The closing of these schools, combined with the continuing marked discrimination against black medical students and physicians in most medical institutions, left a large gap in the supply of black physicians and, by implication, a gap in the provision of health services to the black population. As late as 1947, there were only 588 black medical students, of whom 495 were enrolled at the two remaining schools for black students of medicine (Howard Medical School in Washington, D.C., and Meharry Medical College in Tennessee) and 93 in other schools. [45] While the enrollment of black medical students has increased considerably in recent years, the proportion of black physicians to black population is still low: Whereas 11 percent of the U.S. population is black, only slightly more than 2 percent of all physicians are black. [19] The fact that, in 1975, blacks constituted nearly 7 percent of first-year enrollments in American undergraduate medical-education programs, and 5 percent of enrollments in graduate programs, may represent a first step toward redressing the imbalance with respect to this segment of the American population. [2]

One writer has succinctly put into perspective the primary elements of the movement to reform medical education. By 1914

> the respective roles of the colleges, the universities, the state licensing agencies, and the professional associations crystallized into the forms we still know today. For the first time the societies, licensing associations, and a leading bloc of colleges had common aims: the upgrading of entrance standards to the profession, the specification of curricula in the medical schools, the suppression of the weakest proprietary institutions, and the reduction in the number of students graduating from medical schools. These aims interlocked. The reform movement was partly educational, partly restrictionist, having as its goal both more highly trained and fewer physicians. [45, p. 55]

Specialization. As the reform of undergraduate medical education progressed, enabling the profession to raise its standards and simultaneously to reduce its ranks, specialization in various aspects of medicine began to appear. This was partly the result of the reform movement's drive toward excellence, and partly of the nation's increasing focus on scientific-technological development in all sectors, including the health sector. The social and pecuniary potential of medical specialization (power, prestige, and wealth) soon became evident, and the mad scramble for certification in a specialty that started has continued unabated. As early as 1923 there were twenty-three medical specialties; in 1970 there were sixty-three. In 1923, over 15,000 or 10 percent of physicians listed themselves in the AMA directory as being full-time specialists. By 1931, the number of specialists had risen to 25,000 or 17 percent of active physicians. By 1950, the proportion was over one-third, by 1963 nearly two-thirds, and by 1969 over three-quarters (table 3-3).

Certain specialties grew much more rapidly than others. Table 3-4, which shows an index of growth in the number of full-time medical specialists by field of specialty, shows that the most rapid growth was in anesthesiology, in which nearly seventy times as many physicians were engaged in 1966 as in 1923 (the year when the fewest of all specialists were anesthesiologists). Other specialties experiencing rapid growth were, in order of magnitude, obstetrics/gynecology (twenty times more in 1966 than in 1923), pathology and bacteriology (nineteen times more), and pediatrics and orthopedic surgery (each eighteen times more). The slowest rates of growth were

Table 3-3
Physicians in Active Practice in the United States, by Type of Specialty, Selected Years, 1931-1969

	1931	*1932*	*1949*	*1960*	*1963*	*1969*
			A. Percentage			
N	145 225	156 970	173 129	199 846	223 212	251 150
Total	100	100	100	100	100	100
Part-time specialists and general practitioners	83	76	64	43	35	23
Full-time specialists	17	24	36	57	65	77
Medicine	5	7	11	19	21	24
Surgery[a]	10	13	18	26	29	30
Psychiatry, neurology	1	1	3	5	7	8
Other	1	3	4	7	8	15
			B. Ratio per 10,000 Population			
Total	11.7	11.9	11.6	10.9	11.7	12.5
Part-time specialists and general practitioners	9.7	9.1	7.4	4.7	4.1	2.9
Full-time specialists	2.0	2.8	4.2	6.3	7.7	9.6
Medicine	0.5	0.8	1.3	2.0	2.5	2.9
Surgery[a]	1.2	1.5	2.1	2.9	3.4	3.8
Psychiatry, neurology	0.1	0.2	0.3	0.6	0.8	1.0
Other	0.2	0.3	0.5	0.8	1.0	1.9

Source: R. Stevens, *American Medicine and the Public Interest* (New Haven, Conn. and London: Yale University Press, 1971).

Note: Excludes interns, residents, fellows, and inactive physicians. Includes those in private and non-private practice, both federal and nonfederal.

[a] Includes anesthesiology.

in ophthalmology and otolaryngology, which had been the leading specialties in 1923. Surgery, which held second place in 1923, grew only eight-fold in the forty-three-year period, although in absolute numbers it ranked second to internal medicine in 1966. Between 1923 and 1940, that is, before World War II, public health grew faster than any other specialty; but by 1966 it lagged far behind most others. In general, there were nearly ten times as many specialists in 1966 as in 1923. The fastest growth for most specialties occurred during the postwar period, 1949-1962. What is not clear from the available data on specialization is what role the inflow of foreign physicians after the war played in the rapid growth of certain specialties, such as anesthesiology and pathology, in which foreign physicians are heavily engaged.

As the number of specialists grew, the number of general practitioners declined, partly because specialty practice was viewed as more challenging,

Table 3-4
Index Numbers of Growth in Number of Full-Time Medical Specialists in the United States, by Field of Specialty, Selected Years, 1923-1966

Specialty	*Number in 1923*	*Index Numbers*					*Number in 1966*
		1923	*1940*	*1949*	*1962*	*1966*	
Anesthesiology	107	100	266	1,150	5,191	6,987	7,476
Dermatology, venerology	361	100	270	445	736	821	2,964
Internal medicine	1,958	100	329	638	1,398	1,581	30,948
Obstetrics, gynecology	696	100	366	729	1,678	1,991	13,861
Ophthalmology, otolaryngology	4,703	100	361	196	231	246	11,560
Orthopedic surgery	326	100	331	624	1,497	1,816	5,921
Pathology, bacteriology	317	100	311	546	1,420	1,874	5,941
Pediatrics	689	100	350	626	1,525	1,823	12,558
Psychiatry, neurology	945	100	254	499	1,310	1,611	15,224
Pulmonary diseases	305	100	203	345	382	287	874
Public health, aviation medicine	315	100	494	497	846	626	1,971
Radiology, roentgenology	588	100	270	487	1,090	1,303	7,659
Surgery, occupational medicine	3,336	100	199	362	717	798	25,605
Urology	762	100	226	286	479	536	4,085
All specialties	15,408	100	239	404	832	965	148,628

Source: Based on data in R. Stevens, *American Medicine and the Public Interest* (New Haven, Conn. and London: Yale University Press, 1971).

Notes: Includes specialists in active practice, hospital practice (other than interns and residents), and other forms of practice. Figures for 1966 refer to primary interest rather than to full-time devotion to the specialty. Hospital administration and physical medicine were not recognized specialties until after 1940 and are thus excluded from the table; the former numbered 273 in 1949, 979 in 1962, and 2,620 in 1966, while the latter numbered 234, 632, and 682 for those years, respectively.

and partly because of the accompanying prestige and financial rewards. From table 3-3 it is evident that general practitioners declined not only in absolute numbers (from over 120,000 in 1931 to over 57,000 in 1969), but also as a percentage of the total (from 83 percent in 1931 to 23 percent in 1969), as well as in relation to population (from 9.7 per 10,000 in 1931 to 2.9 per 10,000 in 1969).

As a result of the rise of the specialist and the decline of the general practitioner, severe distribution problems developed. Since medical services are rendered on a personal basis, there are geographic limits beyond which certain types of medical services cannot be exported. The very nature of specialty practice as it evolved over the years has demanded an array of facilities, equipment, and staff concentrated in institutions and geographic areas having particular characteristics. For those segments of the population residing outside the periphery of this concentration of activity, access to secondary and tertiary medical services has been attenuated. With the decline in the number of general practitioners, such populations were not likely to have been compensated by an increase in primary care.

As specialization advanced, the structure of medical education and training changed from one based on a general, standardized, undergraduate education obtained largely in a medical school to one focusing on graduate education, with an increasing array of hospital-based specialty training programs. The history of specialization is thus essentially the history of the rapid rise in the number of trainees (interns and residents) in the hospital setting, with the focus of training shifting to secondary and tertiary care.

There appears to have been no national regulatory or planning mechanism linking the total number of residencies, or their distribution among specialties, to the estimated needs of the nation for medical care, to the number of persons graduating each year from medical schools, or to the specialty interests of graduates. Moreover, there was no system of budgeting that might limit the number of residencies offered, on either a national, regional, hospital, or specialty basis. The task (or the pleasure) of creating residencies was thus left to the specialists in teaching hospitals, the heads of divisions in hospitals, and the heads of departments of medical schools or hospitals. The total number of residencies and internships offered in a given year, and their distribution by specialty, was thus essentially the sum of decisions made in each hospital having the relevant programs. [51]

Such decisions reflected hardly any relationship between the number of internship and residency positions offered, and the number that could reasonably be filled by graduates of American and Canadian medical schools, as is evident in table 3-5 and figure 3-2, which reflect a combination of residencies and internships. On the average, only 62 percent were filled by such graduates during the period 1950–1975. Even with the inclusion of those filled by FMGs, there was a substantial number of unfilled positions each year, 20 percent on the average during the 1950s and 1960s. Between 1950 and 1975 the number of positions offered more than doubled (an increase of 135 percent), while the number filled by graduates of American and Canadian schools increased by 127 percent. In other words, the increase in the number of positions filled by domestic production did not keep pace with the increase in the number of positions offered. This gap was partly filled by FMGs, whose numbers increased eight-fold (by 774 percent) over the twenty-five-year period. This increase in FMG participation was sufficient not only to compensate largely for the gap left by domestic production, but also to bring the number of unfilled positions down from 25 percent of the positions offered in 1950–1951 to 8 percent of those offered in 1974–1975.

During the period 1950–1971, the proportion of offered positions filled by domestic stock declined each year. Beginning in 1973, however, there was a distinct reversal of this trend, so that by 1974–1975 the proportion of places filled by domestic graduates was almost at the same level as that

Table 3–5
AMA-Approved Internships and Residencies, Selected Years, 1950–1975

					Positions Filled by:					
	Total Positions Offered[a] (1)		Total Positions Filled (2)		USMGs[b] (3)		FMGs[c] (4)		Positions Vacant (5)	
Year	*Number*	*Percentage*	*Number*	*Percentage*	*Number*	*Percentage*	*Number*	*Percentage*	*Number*	*Percentage*
1950–1951	28,734	100	21,525	75	19,453	68	2,072	7	7,209	25
1955–1956	38,132	100	31,028	82	24,995	66	6,033	16	7,104	18
1960–1961	45,333	100	37,562	83	27,627	61	9,935	22	7,771	17
1965–1966	51,933	100	41,568	80	30,074	58	11,494	22	10,358	20
1970–1971	61,938	100	51,015	82	34,708	56	16,307	26	10,923	18
1973–1974	66,302	100	60,109	91	41,765	63	18,348	28	5,953	9
1974–1975	67,613	100	62,326	92	44,211	65	18,115	27	5,287	8

Source: American Medical Association, 76th Annual Report, "Medical Education in the United States, 1975–1976," Appendix 1, *Journal of the American Medical Association* 236(1976):3049–3055.

[a] Sum of the residencies and internships.

[b] Includes Canadian graduates.

[c] Includes Americans graduated abroad.

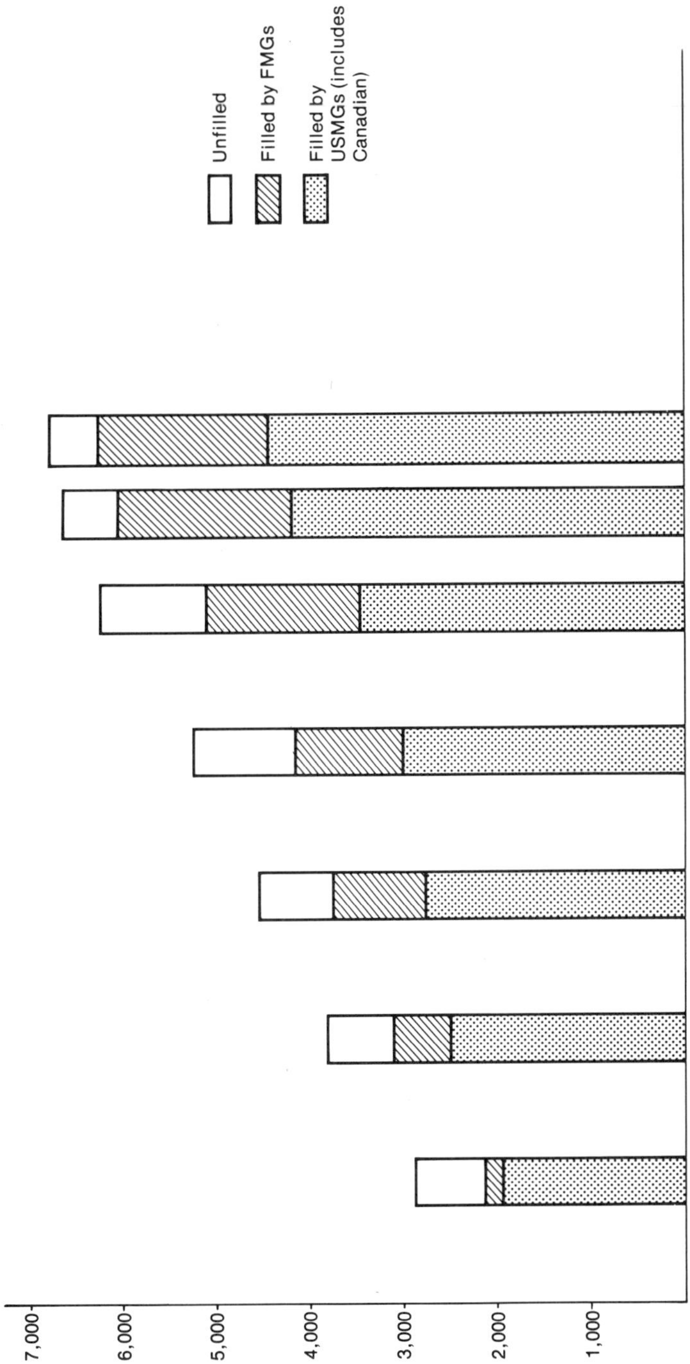

Source: Table 3–5.

Figure 3–2. AMA-Approved Internships and Residencies, 1950–1975.

existing in 1950–1951, that is, before FMGs had started to play any significant role. If the number of places offered and the number filled by domestic graduates continue to increase at the same rate as in recent years, by 1980 there could be 76,000 places offered, all taken by graduates of American and Canadian schools.

With respect to internships, as distinct from residencies and internships combined, a similar pattern developed, but with somewhat different implications. Table 3-6, which compares the number of internships offered with the number of new medical graduates, shows that over the academic years 1965–1966 to 1971–1972, there was a considerable discrepancy between the two factors. This discrepancy reached a peak in 1970–1971, when there were 7,000 or 46 percent more internships offered than there were new graduates. As a result, 3,339 or 22 percent of the positions offered were filled by FMGs and 25 percent were declared unfilled. The two figures do not add to 46 percent because not all new graduates undertake internship. In fact, after 1971–1972 increasing numbers began skipping internship and going straight into residency programs. Accordingly, as seen in table 3-6, hospitals began to reduce their offers of internships; by 1974–1975, the number offered was less by 1,172 or 11 percent than the number of new graduates for the preceding year.

The trend in the types of internship programs offered over the years is of interest. From table 3-7 it can be seen that during the 1960s the propor-

Table 3-6
Number of Internships Offered Relative to Number of Graduates of Medical Schools in the United States, 1956–1975

Year	*Internship Positions Offered (Number)*	*U.S. Graduates of one Year Earlier (Number)*	*Discrepancy (Number)*	*Positions Filled by FMGs (Number)*	*Positions Unfilled (Number)*
1965–1966	12,954	7,409	+5,545	2,361	3,284
1966–1967	13,569	7,574	+5,995	2,793	3,203
1967–1968	13,761	7,743	+6,018	2,913	3,342
1968–1969	14,112	7,973	+6,139	3,270	3,648
1969–1970	15,003	8,059	+6,944	2,939	4,195
1970–1971	15,354	8,367	+6,987	3,339	3,802
1971–1972	15,422	8,974	+6,448	3,946	3,356
1972–1973	13,650	9,551	+4,099	3,924	2,487
1973–1974	12,165	10,391	+1,774	3,425	1,134
1974–1975	10,441	11,613	−1,172	2,756	614

Source: American Medical Association, 76th Annual Report, "Medical Education in the United States 1975–1976," appendix 1, *Journal of the American Medical Association* 236(1976):3049–3055.

Table 3-7
Types of Internship Programs Offered in the United States, 1959–1975

	Type of Program								
	Rotating:								
	No Major Emphasis		Emphasis on a Specialty		Straight		Family and General Practice		Total
Year	Number	Percentage	Number	Percentage	Number	Percentage	Number	Percentage	Number
1959–1960	816	75	33	3	246	22	0	0	1,097
1960–1961	817	70	69	6	276	24	5	[a]	1,167
1961–1962	737	61	107	9	359	30	9	[a]	1,212
1962–1963	697	56	133	11	391	32	14	1	1,235
1963–1964	661	52	153	12	432	34	17	1	1,263
1964–1965	658	50	189	14	467	35	14	1	1,328
1965–1966	641	45	251	17	531	37	17	1	1,440
1966–1967	568	24	1,211	51	582	24	17	[a]	2,378
1967–1968	563	20	1,502	54	687		16	[a]	2,768
1968–1969	581	21	1,504	54	703	25	0	0	2,788
1969–1970	504	17	1,675	57	714	25	29	1	2,922
1970–1971	523	17	1,665	53	963	30	[b]	[b]	3,151
1971–1972	499	15	1,737	53	1,018	31	[b]	[b]	3,254
1972–1973	459	15	1,562	54	892	31	[b]	[b]	2,913
1973–1974	411	19	948	43	835	38	[b]	[b]	2,194
1974–1975	338	19	729	41	719	40	[b]	[b]	1,786

Sources (for 1959–1960 to 1968–1969): American Medical Association, Division of Medical Education, *Directory of Approved Internships and Residences* (Chicago: American Medical Association, various years); (for other years): ibid., 76th Annual Report, "Medical Education in the United States 1975–1976," appendix 1, *Journal of the American Medical Association* 236(1976):3049–3055.

[a] less than 1 percent

[b] beginning with the year 1970–1971, family and general practice were listed as residency programs.

tion of programs offering rotating internships focusing on a specialty rose from 3 to 54 percent of all internship programs offered, while the proportion of those with no particular major focus declined from 75 to 21 percent. The proportion of straight programs (strictly specialist internships in medicine, surgery, pediatrics, and pathology) remained fairly steady, averaging about 28 percent of all programs offered during the decade. While general practice as a specialty was not recognized until 1960, it is nonetheless noteworthy that so few programs were offered in this area over the course of the decade.

The implications for the distribution of medical manpower and services are evident not only in the number of internships and residency positions offered and taken, but also in their distribution by specialty (table 3-8) and by the nature and size of hospital (tables 3-9 and 3-10).

With regard to residencies in terms of specialties (table 3-8), it is interesting to note the growth between 1968 and 1974 in the proportion of filled positions in each specialty. Whereas in 1968 only nine specialties had 90 percent or more of their offered positions filled, by 1974 the number was fifteen. Overall, the proportion of positions filled by domestic graduates was only slightly greater in 1974 than it had been six years earlier (70 percent compared with 68 percent), which in 1974 still left a gap of nearly one-third of all positions, for which domestic graduates were not available. The largest gap was in general practice, where only 13 percent of filled positions in 1974 were taken by domestic graduates—a substantial decline from the 45 percent in 1968. It should be noted, however, that by 1974 a new specialty called "family practice" had been created, and 92 percent of the filled positions in that specialty were taken by domestic graduates. This may explain the decline in general practice, which formerly included family practice. Other areas experiencing a broadening gap included physical medicine, where the proportion of filled positions taken by domestic graduates declined from 60 to 30 percent, and psychiatry, child psychiatry, thoracic surgery, and radiology. Specialties in which significantly increasing proportions of positions were being filled by domestic graduates were colon and rectal surgery, pediatric cardiology, and pediatrics, although the gap left in these areas was still high in 1974. On the other hand, domestic graduates showed a declining interest in psychiatry, thoracic surgery, and otolaryngology, as well as in general practice and physical medicine. Their interest in anesthesiology and pathology, which was only moderate in 1968, declined further in 1974. In both 1968 and 1974 hospitals appeared to have the least difficulty in recruiting domestic graduates to residencies in dermatology, ophthalmology, and orthopedic surgery.

With regard to the distribution of internships and residencies by type of hospital, table 3-9 shows that, whereas in 1960 over one-third of the internships and over half of the residencies offered were in university-affiliated hospitals, by 1970 the proportions reached two-thirds and three-quarters, respectively. Moreover, as shown in table 3-10, domestic graduates in general showed a greater tendency to take residency positions in affiliated than in nonaffiliated hospitals. Within affiliated hospitals, in 1968 they tended more toward those with fewer than 200 beds, their second choice being those with at least 500 beds. In 1974, more were inclining toward those with 200-300 beds. In nonaffiliated hospitals in 1974, domestic graduates were more inclined than in 1968 toward hospitals with fewer than 200 beds and less inclined toward those with at least 500 beds. In all cases, the supply of domestic graduates was insufficient to fill the positions offered, the overall shortage in 1974 being about 30 percent, and the shortage in medium-sized nonaffiliated hospitals being close to 70 percent.

On the whole, the data on internships and residencies reinforce the point that there has been little relationship between the numbers of trainee positions created and the demand for them on the part of domestic graduates. One can only assume that many positions were created with the expectation of their being filled by FMGs. Moreover, it is to be noted that the specialist physician who has several trainees under his guidance has that many more assistants to help with his work and to care for patients admitted to the hospital. Additionally, the salaries of interns and residents are usually charged to the hospital budget which, in turn, helps to determine the daily rate charged to patients. Given that about 90 percent of hospital revenues and about 50 percent of physicians' fees are covered by private health insurance or by government programs, most of the cost of interns and residents is borne by the medical system as a whole, not by the hospital, the medical school, the supervising physician, or the individual hospitalized patient. [51] Thus there has been little incentive on the part of hospitals to control the number of traineeship positions offered.

With the advent of specialization on a large scale, the focus on producing what Flexner had viewed as a standardized "safe general practitioner" was largely deflected. Instead, medical schools were educating for a multitude of possible careers, and the question of medical manpower no longer rested solely on the number of students entering schools, since there was no longer any assurance that one graduate would be similar, as a physician, to another. As a result, the problem of improving the supply of physicians no longer rested solely on increasing the number of medical students, but also depended on the physician's ultimate choice of specialty and location of practice.

Role of the Government. The U.S. government has always been deeply concerned about the nation's health and has made gargantuan efforts to ensure a healthy population—through its programs for the prevention and control of disease; its financing of health research, medical education, and

Table 3–8
Hospital Residencies in the United States, by Specialty, 1968–1974

	Total Positions Filled				Percentage of Positions Filled by			
	Number		Percentage		USMGs[a]		FMG	
Specialty	*1968*	*1974*	*1968*	*1974*	*1968*	*1974*	*1968*	*1974*
Anesthesiology	1,502	2,044	78	90	50	46	50	54
Child psychiatry	473	570	71	77	81	69	19	31
Colonic and rectal surgery	29	30	85	88	44	67	55	33
Dermatology	512	757	95	97	91	92	9	8
General practice	402	286	45	86	45	13	55	87
Internal medicine	6,163	11,024	86	97	65	73	35	27
Neurological surgery	504	607	92	94	78	80	22	20
Neurology	684	1,045	82	93	74	71	26	29
Obstetrics and gynecology	2,503	3,421	87	94	63	67	37	33
Ophthalmology	1,238	1,568	96	99	93	92	7	8
Orthopedic surgery	1,758	2,375	94	97	88	89	12	11
Otolaryngology	873	994	95	95	88	83	12	17
Pathology[b]	2,230	2,903	62	82	52	49	48	51
Pediatrics	2,185	4,784	86	96	58	69	42	31
Pediatric allergology	64	114	75	84	78	80	22	20
Pediatric cardiology	125	124	80	87	47	70	53	30
Physical medicine	277	396	58	78	60	30	40	70
Plastic surgery	201	397	92	94	78	81	22	19
Psychiatry	3,620	4,370	75	87	71	64	29	36
Radiology[c]	2,240	3,160	85	86	80	73	20	27

Surgery	6,064	7,354	90	94	63	68	37	32
Thoracic surgery	279	296	91	93	75	65	25	35
Urology	867	1,117	91	97	75	79	25	21
Total	34,794	49,736	83	93	68	70	32	30
Family practice	—	2,669	—	80	—	92	—	8
Nuclear medicine	—	94	—	73	—	64	—	36

Sources (1968): American Medical Association, Division of Medical Education, *Directory of Approved Internships and Residencies* (Chicago: American Medical Association, various years); (1974): ibid., 76th Annual Report, "Medical Education in the United States 1975-1976," appendix 1, *Journal of the American Medical Association* 236(1976):3049-3055.

Note: Table includes hospital residencies only. Residencies filled outside the hospital numbered 253 in 1968 and 186 in 1974.

[a] USMGs include Canadian graduates.

[b] Pathology includes forensic pathology and neuropathology.

[c] Radiology includes diagnostic and therapeutic radiology.

Table 3-9
Internship and Residency Positions Offered in University-Affiliated Hospitals in the United States, Selected Years, 1960–1974

	Internships			*Residencies*		
Year	*Total Number*	*Number in University-Affiliated Hospitals*	*Percentage in University-Affiliated Hospitals*	*Total Number*	*Number in University-Affiliated Hospitals*	*Percentage in University-Affiliated Hospitals*
1960–1961	12,547	4,779	38	32,620	17,588	54
1962–1963	12,024	5,907	49	36,162	22,373	62
1964–1965	12,728	4,964	39	38,373	18,622	48
1966–1967	13,569	7,615	56	38,895	24,854	64
1968–1969	14,509	8,329	57	42,889	27,208	63
1970–1971	14,683	9,457	64	46,250	35,803	77
1972–1973	12,165	10,489	86	53,688	48,703	91
1974–1975	10,441	9,298	89	57,172	52,805	92

Sources (1974–1975): American Medical Association, 76th Annual Report, "Medical Education in the United States 1975–1976," appendix 1, *Journal of the American Medical Association* 236(1976): 3049-3055; (all other years): ibid., Division of Medical Education, Directory of Approved Internships and Residences (Chicago: American Medical Association, various years).

hospital construction; and its health-insurance schemes (Medicare and Medicaid). Although these efforts have been well intended, the exorbitant costs involved did not effect a commensurate improvement in the basic structure of health-care delivery. If anything, they fostered even greater abuse of the free-enterprise system and exaggerated rather than diminished both the emphasis on costly sophisticated technology and the maldistribution of health personnel, particularly of physicians.

After World War II, the federal government's role in health research grew at an extraordinary pace. Research expenditures from all sources grew from $0.02 per capita in 1940 to $12.50 per capita in 1974, with the public share of expenditures on health research increasing from 66 percent in 1950 to over 90 percent in 1973. Expenditure by the government's National Institutes of Health (NIH) rocketed from $256 million in 1960 to $1,643 million in 1974. Some of this research was carried out at NIH, but most was carried out, through federal grants, at the nation's medical schools and hospitals. [60]

The result was that by 1960 the medical school had become largely a federally dominated research institution, whose purpose was only partly to educate students for the practice of medicine. In 1969, over 272,000 students who were not medical students in the traditional sense were accorded

Table 3–10
Residencies in the United States, by Medical-School Affiliation and Bed Capacity, 1968–1974

	Total Positions Filled				*Percentage of Positions Filled by:*			
	Number		*Percentage*		*USMGs*		*FMGs*	
Hospital Type	*1968*	*1974*	*1968*	*1974*	*1968*	*1974*	*1968*	*1974*
Affiliated								
Combined hospitals	10,741	21,288	89	94	79	79	21	21
Less than 200 beds	609	2,153	80	89	83	72	17	28
200–299 beds	785	1,176	80	88	61	77	39	23
300–499 beds	4,132	7,316	79	90	66	66	34	34
500 or more beds	11,367	16,825	86	92	73	68	27	32
Subtotal	27,634	48,760	85	92	74	73	26	27
Nonaffiliated								
Combined hospitals	1,043	304	77	86	63	54	37	46
Less than 200 beds	388	682	64	79	41	63	59	37
200–299 beds	765	340	73	86	34	28	66	72
300–499 beds	2,072	1,087	70	87	34	35	66	65
500 or more beds	2,892	1,326	76	87	48	37	52	63
Subtotal	7,160	3,739	73	86	44	42	56	58
Total	34,794	52,499	83	92	68	71	32	29

Sources (1968): American Medical Association, Division of Medical Education, *Directory of Approved Internships and Residencies* (Chicago: American Medical Association, various years); (1974): ibid., 76th Annual Report, "Medical Education in the United States 1975–1976," appendix 1, *Journal of American Medical Association* 236(1976):3049–3055.

Note: USMGs include Canadian graduates.

teaching time equivalent to what approximately 55,000 undergraduate medical students would be likely to consume. In the same year, however, there were only about 36,000 undergraduate medical students. Even in terms of full-time student equivalents, nonmedical students outnumbered medical students by a ratio of about three to two. [1] The number of biomedical researchers grew by 192 percent between 1950 and 1970, while the number of domestically trained physicians grew by only 46 percent between 1950 and 1974. In 1969 federal outlays for health-manpower training included $210 million for the training of research personnel, compared with only $170 million for the training of physicians, that is, 29 and 24 percent of federal outlays for health manpower training, respectively. Of the total of federal outlays for health, 9 percent went to research and 1 percent to the training of physicians. [60]

Clearly, therefore, federal subsidies to universities for medical research substantially diverted the interest of teaching staff from their traditional role of providing medical education. Moreover, the trend did not run counter to the interests of the AMA, which supported federal funding of biomedical research in the schools, while opposing federal aid to teaching by the same faculties. As a result, much of the teaching came to be concealed in research budgets, with the salary of the teacher often paid on the representation that he was a full-time or nearly full-time researcher. While the number of full-time faculty had reached some 23,000 by 1969, or an average of over 250 per school (as compared with about 70 per school in 1950 and about 120 in 1960), many, if not most, were not regularly involved in teaching medical students, even though the ratio of faculty to medical students was two to three, and in some schools even one to one. This situation arose largely as a result of the way in which faculty salaries were funded. In 1969 nearly half the faculty received part of their salaries from federal funds, predominantly from funds for research; nearly one-third received the larger part of their salary in this way; and about 15 percent were totally dependent on federal funds. In summary, it was economically to their advantage for faculty to focus on research rather than training. Moreover, through their accumulation of federal grants, principal investigators on the faculties of medical schools were able to create power blocs built around specific and often highly esoteric research projects, leaving to the deans of medical schools the task of coping with the schools' proportionally dwindling general income, part of which had to be used to pay for overhead costs generated by research projects but largely unaccounted for in research grants. [45]

While the sharp focus on research tended to diminish interest in teaching, and thus in the production of physicians, it also tended to promote university-affiliated hospitals at the expense of community hospitals. Moreover, political rather than social considerations played the predominant role in determining the diseases on which research focused. In 1974 nearly one-third of the federal outlay for health research was devoted to research on cancer and on heart and lung diseases, which are particularly alarming to white middle-class males. Mental illness, which ranks third among causes of days of hospitalization and fourth among causes of limitation of activity, received only 6 percent of this outlay. Only 7 percent went for research on arthritis and metabolic and digestive disorders, which together are the leading causes of days of hospitalization. Moreover, the proportion of people whose activities are limited by arthritis is far greater among those with low incomes than among those with high incomes. [60] The biased nature of research in turn effected a bias in the focus of medical education, the products of which could hardly avoid being biased in their choices of what, and therefore whom, to treat. Such biases created shortages of medical services in areas of need.

Federal research grants to medical schools favored not only particular types of schools and diseases, but also particular geographic areas. In 1970 the federal government provided a billion dollars to medical and other health-professional schools, or an average of nearly $84,000 per medical-school graduate. This program strongly favored states that were already rich in physicians. Of the twelve medical schools receiving the largest portion of total federal grants to medical schools, six are located in New York, Massachusetts, and California—the states with the highest number of physicians per unit of population. In 1970 the ten states having the highest proportion of federal grants to medical schools per graduate had a combined ratio of 16 physicians per 10,000 population—almost 50 percent higher than that for the ten states receiving the lowest proportion of grants. In 1970 grants to the top ten schools averaged $208,000 per graduate, compared with an average of $56,000 per graduate for the bottom ten schools. [19]

In 1974 over half of all federal expenditures for health were expressed in the form of Medicare and Medicaid, two programs created in 1965 to finance health care for the aged and the medically indigent, respectively. With respect to Medicare, there seems to be little doubt that it has effected improvements in the quality and quantity of care received by the elderly. However, its benefits appear to have accrued largely to the urban population to the detriment of rural dwellers, for whom the premium for Medicare is the same as it is for urban people. In the sixteen states having the lowest average monthly reimbursements for medical services, the populations are predominantly rural. [60]

Medicare and Medicaid payments have been disproportionately high for states with high physician coverage per unit of population, and disproportionately low for those with low coverage. As was the case with federal research grants, New York, Massachusetts, and California (the three states with the highest physician/population ratios) received half of all the nation's Medicaid funds and almost one-third of all Medicare payments, even though less than one-fifth of the nation's people eligible for Medicare and/or Medicaid reside in those states. The following is a comparison of Medicaid payments per inhabitant and Medicare payments per enrollee, for the three states having the highest number of physicians per 10,000 population and for the three states having the lowest number. [19]

State	*Physician/ Population Ratio*	*Medicaid Payments per Capita (dollars)*	*Medicare Payments per Enrollee (dollars)*
Highest ratios			
New York	23.6	66	414
Massachusetts	19.6	47	415
California	19.1	50	478
Lowest ratios			
Mississippi	8.3	4	251
South Dakota	8.0	13	278
Alaska	6.8	9	246
United States	14.8	24	344

This table shows, among other things, that in New York, the state with the highest physician coverage, Medicaid payments per capita in 1970 were nearly three times the national average, while in Mississippi, with only about one-third of the physician coverage obtaining in New York, such payments were only one-sixth of the national average. In other words, New York received sixteen times as much Medicaid per capita as did Mississippi. It also received nearly twice as high Medicare payments per enrollee.

Theoretically, Medicaid was intended to help the poorest segments of America's population. Had it succeeded in this respect, one would expect to find a strong correlation between the percentage of persons in need—those below the poverty level—and the amount of Medicaid payments per inhabitant. In fact, however, the reverse occurred. [19, 55]

	Medicaid Payments per Inhabitant		*Inhabitants below Low-Income Level*	
State	*Amount (dollars)*	*As Percentage of Average in United States*	*Percentage*	*As Percentage of Average in United States*
Least in need				
New York	66	275	11	81
Massachusetts	47	196	9	63
California	50	208	11	81

Most in need				
Mississippi	4	17	35	258
South Dakota	13	54	19	136
Alaska	9	37	13	92
United States	24	100	14	100

It has been hypothesized that discriminatory federal spending encourages the migration of physicians within the United States; that, for example, more Illinois-trained physicians go to California than stay in Illinois, not only because of the climate and other attractions of California, but also because California receives three times more federal aid per graduate than Illinois, two-and-a-half times as much in Medicaid payments, and one-third more in Medicare payments. [19]

Imbalance between Demand and Supply

Given the powerful forces stimulating the demand for medical services on the one hand, and, on the other hand, the equally powerful forces controlling the total supply of domestically trained physicians and conditioning their distribution geographically, institutionally, and with respect to specialty, it is not surprising that a gross imbalance between supply and demand developed in the United States.

The evolution of this imbalance over the period 1950-1974 is depicted in figures 3-3, 3-4, and 3-5:

1. figure 3-3 shows the relative rates of growth in physician supply, population, and real GNP; it is based on table 3-11, which provides data derived from basic information in table 3-12.
2. figure 3-4 shows the relative rates of growth in the number of physicians per 10,000 population, physician earnings per physician, and GNP per capita; it is also based on table 3-11.
3. figure 3-5 shows the growth in the number of new licenses granted for practice in the United States, and is based on data that appear in table 3-13.

In summary, the data show that, in the years following World War II, the supply of physicians lagged behind the demand for medical services. During the period 1950-1960, the increase in the number of physicians only kept pace with the increase in population. The number of physicians (including inactive ones) per 10,000 population remained at about 14.0 for the whole decade, despite the fact that real GNP per capita increased by 21 percent over the decade. During the 1960-1970 period, in which the United

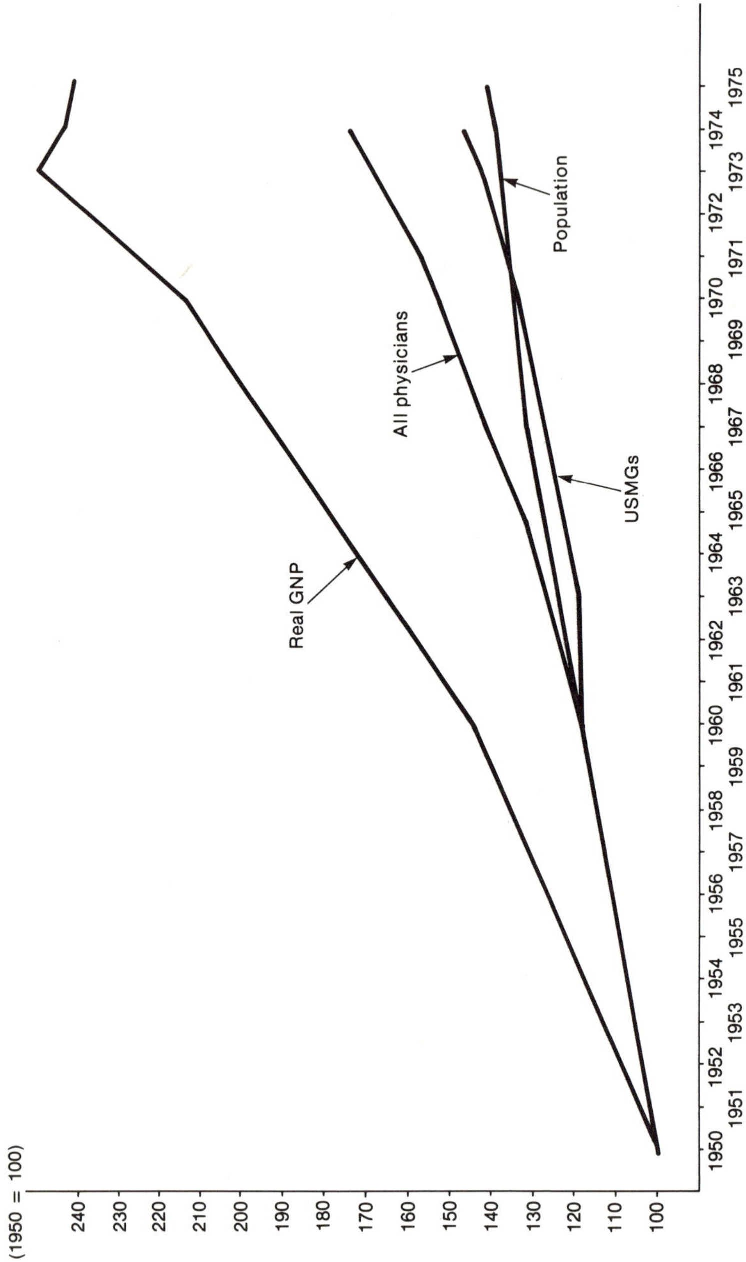

Source: Table 3-11.

Figure 3-3. Relative Growth in Population, Physician Supply, and GNP in the United States, 1950-1975.

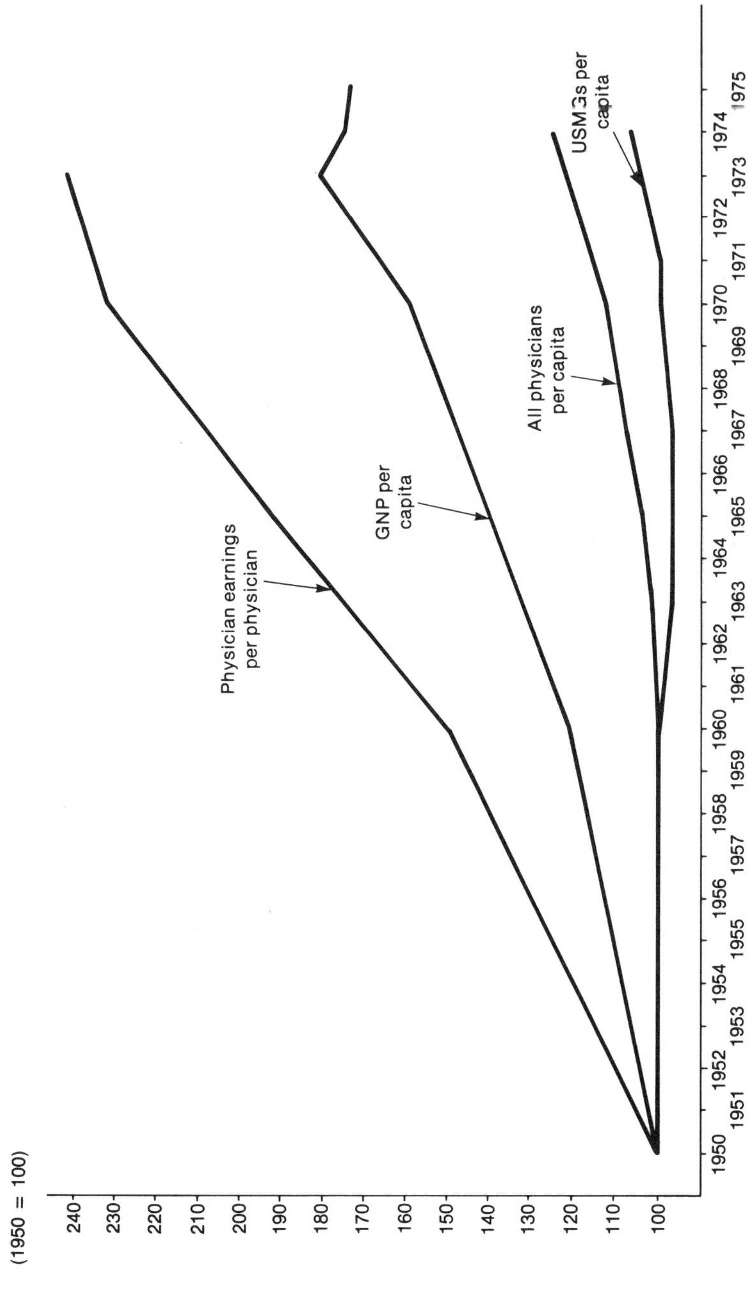

Source: Table 3-11.

Figure 3-4. Relative Growth in Physicians per Capita, Physician Earnings per Physician, and GNP per Capita in the United States, 1950–1975.

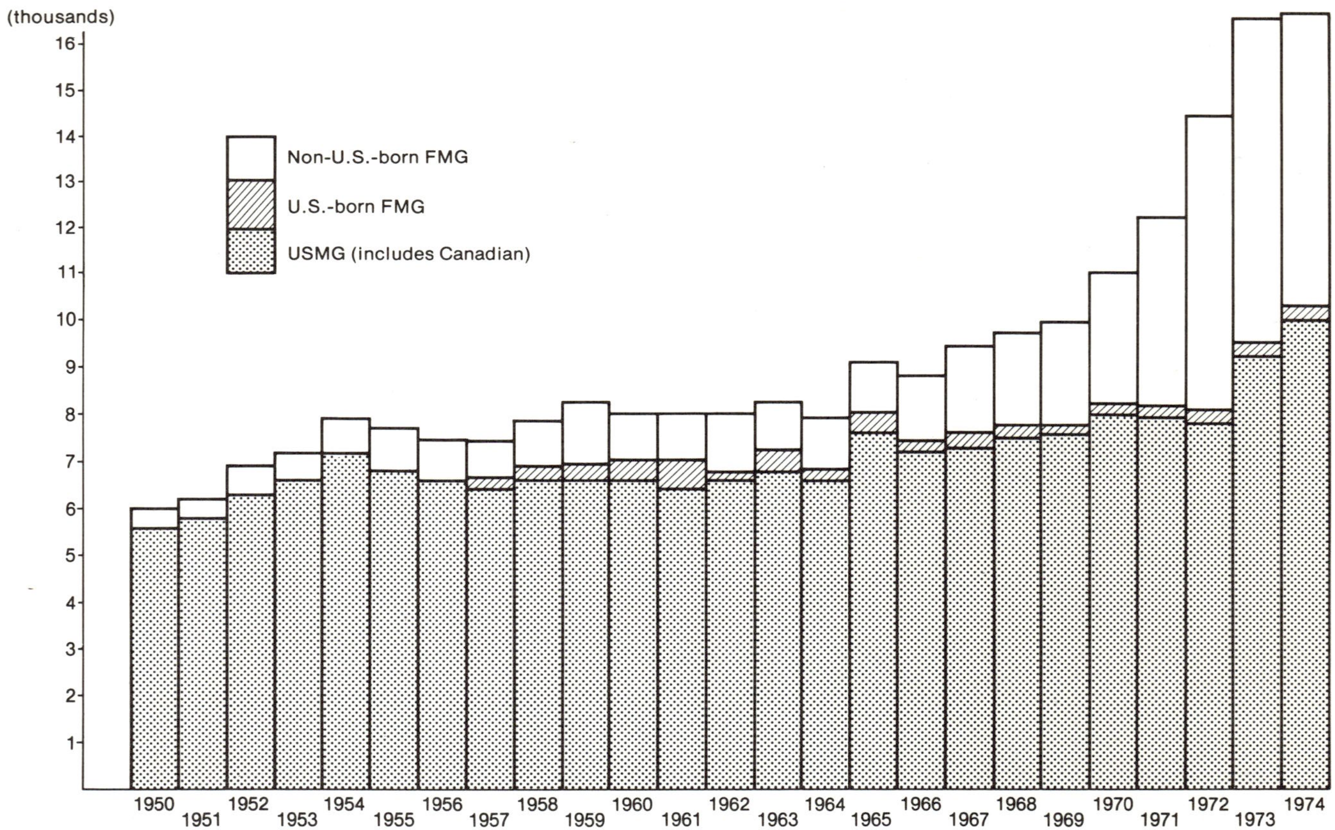

Source: Table 3-13.

Figure 3-5. New Licentiates Representing Additions to the Medical Profession in the United States, by Country of Graduation, 1950-1974.

Table 3-11
Rates of Growth in Population, Physician Supply, GNP, and Physician Earnings in the United States, 1950-1975, Expressed as Index Numbers

	Total Rates				Rates per Capita			
		Number of Physicians			Number of Physicians			
Year	Population (a)	USMGs (b)	All (c)	GNP at 1950 Prices (d)	All (e)	USMGs (f)	GNP at 1950 Prices (g)	Physician Earnings per Active Nonhospital Physician at 1950 Prices (h)
1950	100	100	100	100	100	100	100	100
1960	118	118	118	144	100	121	121	150
1963	123E[a]	119	126		101	96		
1965	127		132		104			193
1967	131	126	140		108	97		
1970	134	133	152	213	113	100	159	233
1971	135	136	156		116	100		
1972	136		162		119			
1973	137	142	167	248	121	104	181	242
1974	138	146	173	242	125	106	175	
1975	139			241			174	

Sources: Based on table 3-12 and derived as follows (column numbers refer to those in table 3-12): column a—column 8; column b—column 1 – column 2; column c—column 1; column d—column 9 ÷ column 11; column e—column 13; column f—column 14; column g—column 12; column h—column 7 ÷ column 11.

[a] E = estimate.

Table 3–12
Basic Data Used to Calculate Index Numbers in Table 3–11

Year	*Total Physicians (Number) (1)*	*FMGs Including Canadians (Number) (2)*	*Active Physicians (Number) (3)*	*Interns and Residents (Number) (4)*	*Active Nonhospital Physicians (Number) (5)*	*Expenditure on Physician Services ($ million) (6)*	*Expenditure per Active Nonhospital Physician ($) (7)*
1950	219,997	17,000 E[a]	208,997	21,525	187,472	2,747	14,652
1960	260,484	21,000 E	247,257	37,562	209,695	5,684	27,106
1963	276,475	36,569					
1965	292,088		277,575	41,568	236,007	8,745	37,054
1967	308,630	51,866					
1970	334,028	63,391	311,203	51,015	260,188	14,306	54,983
1971	344,823	69,188					
1972	356,534						
1973	366,379	77,660	338,111	60,113	277,998	18,200	65,468
1974	379,748	82,916	350,609				

Year	*Population of United States (Millions) (8)*	*GNP ($ Million) (9)*	*GNP per Capita ($) (10)*	*Consumer Price Index (1950 = 100) (11)*	*GNP per Capita at 1950 Prices (12)*	*Physicians per 10,000 Population: All (13)*	*Physicians per 10,000 Population: USMGs only (14)*
1960	185.4	503,734	2,717	123	2,209	14.0	12.9
1963	194.2			127		14.2	12.4
1965	199.3			131		14.7	
1967	203.7			139		15.2	12.6

1970	209.5	977,080	4,664	161	2,897	15.9	12.9
1971	211.6			168		16.3	13.0
1972	213.0			173		16.7	
1973	214.6	1,303,564	6.088	185	3,291	17.1	13.4
1974	216.3	1,413,206	6,534	205	3,187	17.6	13.7
1975	217.0 E	1,516,338	6,990 E	221	3,163		

Sources: Estimates of early years are based on data in United States Department of Health, Education, and Welfare, Public Health Service, Health Resources Administration, Bureau of Health Resources Development, *The Supply of Health Manpower: 1970 Profiles and Projections to 1990*, DHEW Publication no. HRA 75-38 (Washington, D.C.: U.S. Department of Health, Education, and Welfare, 1974); (column 1, 1963 and 1967): Association of American Medical Colleges, *Graduates of Foreign Medical Schools in the United States: A Challenge to Medical Education* (Washington, D.C.: Association of American Medical Colleges, 1974); (column 1, all other years): United States Department of Health, Education, and Welfare, Public Health Service, Health Resources Administration, National Center for Health Statistics, *Health Resources Statistics Reported from the National Center for Health Statistics 1975* (Rockville, Md.: U.S. Department of Health, Education, and Welfare, 1976); (column 2): table 1-1; (column 3): United States Department of Health, Education, and Welfare, *Health Resources Statistics*; (column 4): American Medical Association, 76th Annual Report, "Medical Education in the United States 1975-1976," appendix 1, *Journal of the American Medical Association* 236(1976):3049-3055; (column 5): column 2 – column 4; (column 6): United States Department of Commerce, Bureau of the Census, *Statistical Abstract of the United States, 1975: National Data Book and Guide to Sources* (Washington, D.C.: U.S. Department of Commerce, 1976); (column 7) column 6 – column 4; (column 8): United States Department of Health, Education, and Welfare, *Health Resources Statistics;* (column 9): *World Almanac and Book of Facts 1977* (New York and Cleveland: Newspaper Enterprise Association, 1976); (column 10): column 9 ÷ column 8; (column 11): United States Department of Commerce, *Statistical Abstract of the United States, 1975;* (column 12): column 10 ÷ column 11; (column 13): column 1 ÷ column 8; (column 14): (column 1 – column 2) ÷ column 8.

[a]E = estimate.

Table 3-13
New Licentiates Representing Additions to the Medical Profession in the United States, by Country of Graduation, 1950-1974

			FMGs		*Total FMGs as Percentage of Total New Licentiates*
Year	*Total (1)*	*U.S. and Canadian (2)*	*Total (3)*	*U.S.-Born (4)*[a]	*(5)*
1950	6,002	5,694	308	—	5
1951	6,273	5,823	450	—	7
1952	6,885	6,316	569	—	8
1953	7,276	6,591	685	—	9
1954	7,917	7,145	772	—	10
1955	7,737	6,830	907	—	11
1956	7,463	6,611	852	—	11
1957	7,455	6,441	1,014	212	14
1958	7,809	6,643	1,166	284	15
1959	8,269	6,643	1,626	366	20
1960	8,030	6,611	1,419	386	18
1961	8,023	6,443	1,580	468	20
1962	8,005	6,648	1,357	201	17
1963	8,283	6,832	1,451	395	17
1964	7,911	6,605	1,306	200	16
1965	9,147	7,619	1,528	411	17
1966	8,851	7,217	1,634	252	18
1967	9,424	7,267	2,157	279	23
1968	9,766	7,581	2,185	235	22
1969	9,978	7,671	2,307	179	23
1970	11,032	8,016	3,016	198	27
1971	12,257	7,943	4,314	210	35
1972	14,476	7,815	6,661	240	46
1973	16,689	9,270	7,419	250 E[b]	44
1974	16,706	10,093	6,613	250 E	40

Sources (1973 and 1974): American Medical Association, 76th Annual Report, "Medical Education in the United States 1975-1976," appendix 1, *Journal of the American Medical Association* 236(1976):3049-3055; (other years): K.N. Williams and B.A. Lockett, "Migration of Foreign Physicians to the United States: The Perspective of Health Manpower Planning," *International Journal of Health Services* 4(1974):213-243.

[a] Column 4—Data not available for years 1950-1956, 1973, and 1974.

[b] E = estimate.

States experienced a vast economic expansion, real GNP rose at an unprecedented rate, increasing by 31 percent. However, the population coverage assured by domestically trained physicians still did not increase. However, because restrictions on the entry of FMGs to the United States were relaxed after 1965, the physician pool was augmented by some 40,000 FMGs. This influx caused the growth in the physician/population ratio to reach 13 percent for the decade 1960–1970. While this growth was still less than that of real GNP per capita, it reflected an improvement in the balance between supply and demand.

The next five years, however, were recession years, and the growth in real GNP per capita slowed down to 9 percent (equivalent to 20 percent for a decade). By that time, however, the increase in the supply of domestically trained physicians was at last beginning to make itself felt; some 35,000 were added to the pool as new licentiates during the four-year period 1970–1974 (figure 3–5 and table 3–13). Thus, during that period the ratio of domestically trained physicians to population grew by 6 percent (equivalent to 21 percent for a decade) and accordingly kept pace with the growth of real GNP per capita. Moreover, the total physician pool was swollen by the addition of some 19,300 FMGs during that period. This additional influx caused the physician/population ratio to increase by 11 percent during that period (equivalent to 29 percent for a decade). Thus, the rate of growth in supply was keeping up with the rate of growth in GNP, but a lot of catching up was still needed to compensate for the low supply in previous years.

It is obvious that, if growth in the domestic production of physicians continues as it has during the period 1970–1974 (first year enrollments in 1975 were 75 percent above those in 1965), there will soon be no need for FMGs, or at least not for additional ones.

This conclusion is based on the assumption that per-capita consumption of physician services (and hence the number of physicians per 10,000 population) grows proportionately with GNP per capita. This can be disputed, however, the main question being whether an individual, when his income increases, still spends the same proportion of income on physician services. The answer probably depends on whether, prior to the increase, the individual was already able to buy all the physician services he needed (perceived himself to need), that is, how affluent he was before. If, as a result of an increase in GNP per capita many people can buy physician services they could not previously afford, they may, collectively, cause an increase in the proportion of total national income spent on health.

Whether or not an increase in GNP per capita provokes an equal increase in the money spent on physician services depends on the elasticity of demand in relation to income. If expenditure on health is any indicator, it would seem that such elasticity is great and that, in fact, increases in income provoke a greater-than-proportional increase in health expenditure. Evidence for this lies in the fact that, while total expenditure on health accounted for only 4.6 percent of GNP in 1970 and 7.7 percent in 1974, expenditure on "personal health care" accounted for 4.0 percent of GNP in 1950, 6.2 percent in 1970, and 6.7 percent in 1974. [55]

This points to the notion that, in a free market, an increase of 75 percent in real GNP per capita for the period 1950–1974 should have provoked an equal or greater increase in the amount of physician services demanded, and hence in the number of physicians required. A commensurate increase of 75 percent in the ratio of domestically trained physicians per 10,000 population would have meant a ratio of 24.5 in 1974, whereas the actual ratio assured that year by such physicians was 13.7. This would have meant a potential gap of about 10.9 physicians per 10,000 population or, in absolute terms, a shortage of 236,000 domestically trained physicians. The 83,000 FMGs in the United States in 1974 had been pulled in by this vacuum.

The second effect of too much money chasing too few physicians was a rise in physician earnings in relation to the average national income. Thus, $18,200 million was spent on physician services ($65,500 per active nonhospital physician) in 1973, compared with $2,744 million (that is, $14,700 per active nonhospital physician) in 1950. This represented an average increase of 346 percent in income per physician, compared with an increase, over the same period, of 235 percent in GNP per capita (at actual, not constant, prices).

Forces in the Donor Countries

Many theories have been put forward as to why people leave their countries, and why they choose certain countries of destination rather than others. In this chapter an attempt has been made to outline in broad terms the interplay of the overall political, social, and economic forces that condition migration, and to analyze in greater detail the powerful forces in the United States that pulled in by far the greatest proportion of migrant physicians. As indicated earlier, however, a large-scale outflow from any individual country will not occur, despite the attractions or need of another country, unless equally powerful pushing forces exist in the homeland.

In the WHO multinational study it was found that most physicians from many countries did not respond to the pull of the United States, or, for that matter, any other country. This can be explained partly by the legal barriers set up at various times at either end, or at both ends, of the potential migratory axis; but other factors also play a role when a free-market situation exists.

Earlier in this chapter, migration was metaphorically represented by the liquid in a pipeline, with the liquid flowing (or sometimes not flowing) in response to the differential pressures of certain factors operating at each end of the pipe. In the context of this analogy, variations in the migration behavior of physicians in response to a given factor can perhaps best be illustrated in the following way, using the United States as the potential recipient of physicians; countries X, Y, and Z as the potential donors; and the production of physicians as the potential factor conditioning the migration of physicians. Thus the United States produces far fewer physicians than it can economically afford, and it has a large effective demand for physicians, but:

1. Country X produces more physicians than it can afford to employ; and many of them migrate to the United States, most probably because they perceive the employment situation as being less favorable at home than in the United States, but perhaps for other reasons.
2. Country Y also produces more physicians than it can afford to employ, but its physicians, even at the risk of unemployment in their profession, prefer to stay at home because they perceive the overall situation as being more favorable in their homeland than in the United States when other important factors are taken into consideration. One such factor could well be family and community ties at home.
3. Country Z, like the United States, also produces fewer physicians than it can afford to employ (that is, the production factor exerts equal pressure at each end of the pipeline, and therefore would not be expected to play a role), but a number of physicians still migrate to the United States because of other factors that are less favorable at home than in the United States. For example, the political situation, or even the work situation, may be less palatable in the home country.

The production factor was used in this illustration because, as was found in the WHO multinational study, imbalances between the supply of physicians and the demand for them (and therefore the rate of production of physicians) appeared to play a very strong role, certainly as a pull factor in the United States and also as a push factor in most, though not all, donor countries. As was shown earlier in this chapter, in some countries political upheavals played an important role in the outflow. Moreover, given the many thousands of physicians in the world who did not migrate, it can be assumed that relatively benevolent forces (as viewed by the physicians themselves), or in some instances perhaps restrictive forces, in the country concerned enabled it to retain its physicians.

What follows is a summary, under various headings, of findings from the WHO multinational study that point up those factors that fostered physician migration generally (rather than specifically to the United States) and those that facilitated the migration. The findings are based on a sample of forty countries, including countries at varying levels of development, having varying political, social, and economic systems, reflecting varying geographic areas, and experiencing varying levels of emigration and/or immigration.

The Role of Development

Above and beyond any pushing and pulling forces that either individually or in combination influence physician migration, there is the overall problem of unequal development. The nature of this inequality was briefly described in the first part of this chapter. In this section, its relationship to physician migration is described.

Using GDP per capita as an indicator of level of affluence, and the number of emigrant (and conversely immigrant) physicians relative to domestic stock as an indicator of percentage loss (and gain) of physicians, the WHO multinational study found that the biggest losses, as well as the biggest gains, were sustained by the developing countries and, within that group, by those at the lower end of the development scale. More generally, it was shown that—given the presence of push or pull factors—the poorer the country, the greater its losses or gains. A poor country subject to push factors risks losing a larger proportion of its physicians than does a richer country under the same circumstances.

The relationship between poverty and size of loss held over the complete range of GDP per capita covered (from $97 to $4,789 in 1970). The same relationship held for recipient countries, but instead of their reflecting gains along a continuum, the recipient countries fell into two distinct categories: poor recipients and rich developed recipients. For the poor recipients (mostly former colonies that did not have enough native-born physicians to replace the departed foreign stock, and/or countries without medical schools), the gains tended to be very high. As for the rich developed recipients (whose GDP per capita of $2,000 or more tended to exert a net pull on physicians), only a few of these experienced net emigration, although a number, mostly Commonwealth nations, had both inflows and outflows.

While an analysis such as the above demonstrates the magnitude of the risks of migration for countries at various levels of affluence, it does not in any way explain why some countries lose physicians while others at the same level of affluence do not. The sections that follow aim to throw some light on this aspect. The forty countries on which most of the subsequent sections are based are shown in table 3-14, grouped by level of GDP per capita (1970) and by migration experience.

The Role of Imbalances between Supply and Demand

The analysis that follows purports to show the relationship between the migration of physicians, the supply of physicians, and the economic base needed to generate the demand for their services.

Table 3-14
Percentage of Physician-Stock Gained, and Percentage Lost through Migration, in a Sample of Countries Grouped according to GDP per Capita in 1970

GDP Group	*Country*	*Percentage Gained*	*Percentage Lost*	*Percentage Net Gain (+) or Loss (−)*
A. GDP less than $800	Brazil		1.4	−1.4
	Cameroon, U. Rep. of	70.2	7.1	+63.1
	China			
	Colombia	3.0 E[a]	12.1	−8.1
	Egypt		13.1	−13.1
	Ethiopia	94.9	0.3	+94.6
	Gabon	87.5	7.3	+80.2
	Haiti		129.6	−129.6
	India		13.0	−13.0
	Indonesia	2.2	5.4	−3.2
	Iran	0.7	39.2	−38.5
	Jamaica	30.6 E	21.4	+9.2
	Korea, Rep. of	0.3	18.8	−18.5
	Lebanon	7.4	40.7	−33.3
	Mauritius	3.6	75.4	−71.8
	Nigeria	38.2	32.2	+6.0
	Pakistan and Bangladesh	4.0 E	15.8	−11.8
	Philippines		67.5	−67.5
	Portugal	0.9	3.2	−2.3
	Saudi Arabia	43.9 G[b]	0.0	+43.9
	Sri Lanka		26.8	−26.8
	Sudan	5.0	5.0	0.0
	Thailand	3.6	29.9	−26.3
	Uruguay		3.0	−3.0
	Yemen	40.8	0.4	+40.4
	Yugoslavia		6.8	−6.8
B. GDP $800 to $2,000	Greece		11.4	−11.4
	Ireland		120.8	−120.8
	Romania		1.7	−1.7
	Venezuela		2.7	−2.7

[a] E = estimation.

[b] G = government employees.

Table 3-14 continued

GDP Group	*Country*	*Percentage Gained*	*Percentage Lost*	*Percentage Net Gain (+) or Loss (−)*
C. GDP over $2,000	Australia	24.4	12.5	+11.9
	Austria	4.1	14.5	−10.4
	Canada	31.2	18.6	+12.6
	Germany, Fed. Rep. of	5.1	4.2	+0.9
	Israel	25.9 E	5.9	+20.0
	Japan	0.6	0.9	−0.3
	New Zealand	27.2	22.3	+4.8
	Sweden	5.0	1.2	+3.8
	United Kingdom	25.7	10.2	+15.5
	United States	21.8 E	0.4	+21.4

Source: World Health Organization, *Multinational Study of the International Migration of Physicians and Nurses: Statistical Enquiry* (unpublished information).

The number of physicians that a country can sustain, that is, those for whom it can provide satisfactory employment, depends largely on that country's level of affluence and to a lesser extent on how the national income is distributed among the various segments of the population and the various economic sectors. The relationship between affluence, expressed as gross domestic product (GDP) per capita, and physician coverage, expressed as the number of physicians per 10,000 population, is illustrated in figure 3-6, which shows thirty-nine of the forty countries plotted on a log-log scale according to these two parameters, together with a regression line fitted to the points. When the migration behavior of each of the countries was compared with their position vis-à-vis the regression line, it was seen that countries to the right of the line tended to lose physicians and those to the left of the line tended to gain physicians. It was concluded therefore that the mathematical relationship between GDP per capita and physician coverage (which expressed the physician coverage as an exponential function of GDP) could be used as a predictor of migration behavior in that it seemed to be an indicator of the level of physician coverage appropriate for each level of GDP—the "sustainable level."

Restating the theory in more specific terms, and assuming that the level of physician supply as determined by the line represents the sustainable level, one would expect countries with a level higher than this sustainable level to suffer an outflow of physicians (actually an overflow, in this case, as distinct from a drain). Conversely, countries with a level lower than the sustainable level would be expected to experience an inflow of foreign physicians.

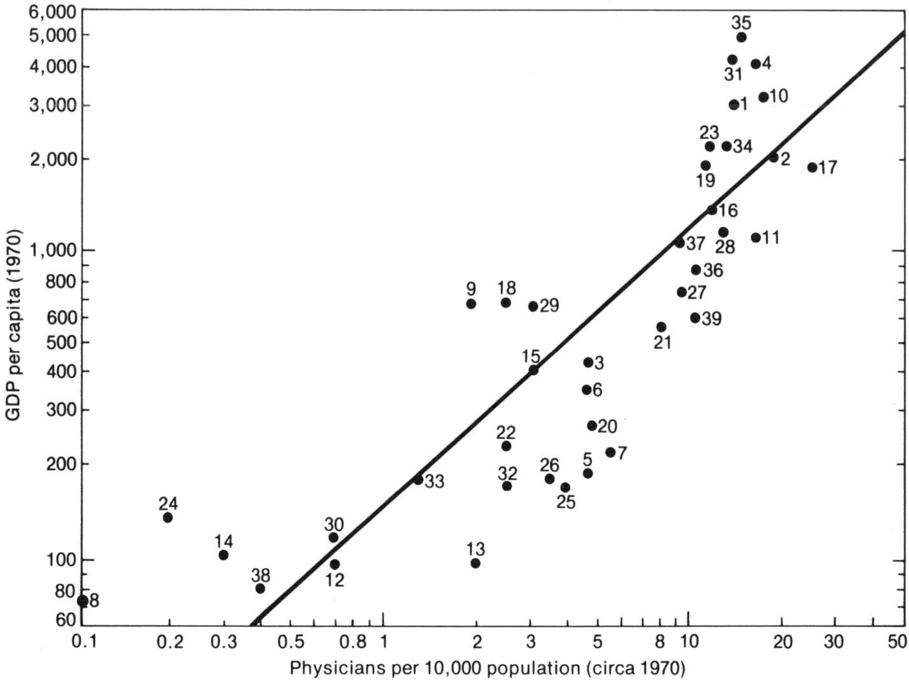

1 Australia
2 Austria
3 Brazil
4 Canada
5 Cameroon; U.Rep. of
6 Colombia
7 Egypt
8 Ethiopia
9 Gabon
10 German Fed. Rep.
11 Greece
12 Haiti
13 India
14 Indonesia
15 Iran
16 Ireland
17 Israel
18 Jamaica
19 Japan
20 Korea, Rep. of
21 Lebanon
22 Mauritius
23 New Zealand
24 Nigeria
25 Pakistan
26 Philippines
27 Portugal
28 Romania
29 S. Arabia
30 Sudan
31 Sweden
32 Sri Lanka
33 Thailand
34 United Kingdom
35 United States
36 Uruguay
37 Venezuela
38 Yemen
39 Yugoslavia
No data on China

Figure 3–6. Gross Domestic Product (GDP) per Capita and Physician Coverage.

In table 3–15 it can be seen that India, for example, which on the basis of this reasoning was able to sustain only 0.6 physicians per 10,000 population in 1970, actually had 2.1 that year—an excess of 1.5 per 10,000 population or, in absolute numbers, an excess of 81,900 physicians. Unless India's economic and political system is exceptional, one would expect India to lose many physicians through migration. On the same assumption, one would expect other countries with an excess of physicians in this context to suffer an outflow. Conversely, countries with a shortage would be expected to

Table 3-15
Differences between Actual and Sustainable Number of Physicians per 10,000 Population, in Countries Grouped according to GDP per Capita in 1970

		Physicians per 10,000 Population		
GDP Group	*Country (1)*	*Actual (2)*	*Sustainable (3)*	*Excess (+) or Shortage (−) (2 − 3) (4)*
A. GDP less than $800	Brazil	4.6	3.2	+1.4
	Cameroon, U. Rep. of	0.4	1.6	−1.4
	China			
	Colombia	4.6	2.6	+2.0
	Egypt	5.5	1.6	+3.9
	Ethiopia	0.1	0.5	−0.4
	Gabon	1.9	5.5	−3.6
	Haiti	0.7	0.6	+0.1
	India	2.1	0.6	+1.5
	Indonesia	0.3	0.7	−0.4
	Iran	3.1	3.1	0.0
	Jamaica	2.5	5.2	−2.7
	Korea, Rep. of	4.8	1.9	+2.9
	Lebanon	8.1	4.4	+3.7
	Mauritius	2.5	1.6	+0.9
	Nigeria	0.2	0.9	−0.7
	Pakistan and Bangladesh	3.9	1.2	+2.7
	Philippines	3.5	1.3	+2.2
	Portugal	9.5	6.0	+3.5
	Saudi Arabia	3.0	5.3	−2.3
	Sri Lanka	2.5	1.2	+1.3
	Sudan	0.7	0.7	0.0
	Thailand	1.3	1.2	+0.1
	Uruguay	10.7	7.0	+3.7
	Yemen	0.4	0.5	−0.1
	Yugoslavia	10.5	5.1	+5.4
B. GDP $800 to $2,000	Greece	16.7	9.0	+7.7
	Ireland	11.8	11.0	+0.8
	Romania	13.1	9.0	+4.1
	Venezuela	9.3	8.6	+0.7

Table 3-15 continued

		Physicians per 10,000 Population		
GDP Group	*Country (1)*	*Actual (2)*	*Sustainable (3)*	*Excess (+) or Shortage (−) (2 − 3) (4)*
C. GDP over $2,000	Australia	13.8	26.5	−12.7
	Austria	18.6	17.0	+1.6
	Canada	16.5	38.0	−21.5
	Germany, Fed. Rep. of	17.7	29.0	−11.3
	Israel	25.1	15.5	+9.6
	Japan	11.4	16.1	−4.7
	New Zealand	11.7	19.5	−7.8
	Sweden	13.8	40.0	−26.2
	United Kingdom	13.3	18.5	−5.2
	United States	15.5	49.0	−33.5

Source (column 2): World Health Organization, *World Health Statistics Annual 1972*, vol. 3 (Geneva: World Health Organization, 1976).

experience an inflow of foreign physicians. Table 3-16 shows, for thirty-nine of the sample of forty countries, the *expected* direction of migration (net inflow or net outflow) together with the *actual* direction of flow as observed. In thirty-five (90 percent) of the countries, the direction of physician migration was as expected. The relationship seems to hold for developing and developed countries alike. At one end of the development scale, for example, the United Republic of Cameroon, one of the countries with a lower level of physician supply than was the average for countries having an equivalent GDP per capita, experienced a net inflow, while India, with a higher than average level, experienced an outflow. At the other end of the development scale, the United Kingdom, with a lower than average level, experienced a net inflow, while Austria, with a higher than average level, experienced a net outflow.

It would therefore seem that, other things being equal, there is a certain sustainable level of physician supply appropriate for each GDP level, and that those countries in which the sustainable level is exceeded invite the risk of physician overflow unless other things are made unequal, that is, unless definite measures are taken to counteract the influence of the economic factors. Whether such measures exist (short of a complete reallocation of resources) is a matter that needs further exploration. As a step in this direction, it would be important to look more closely at the four countries where

Table 3-16
Differences between Actual and Sustainable Numbers of Physicians, and Expected Direction of Physician Migration together with Actual Direction, as Observed in Countries Grouped according to GDP per Capita in 1970

		Stock of Physicians (thousands)			*Direction of Migration*	
GDP Group	*Country (1)*	*Actual (2)*	*Sustainable (3)*	*Excess (+) or shortage (−) (2 − 3) (4)*	*Expected (5)*	*Actual (6)*
A. GDP less than $800	Brazil	46.1	31.6	+14.5	Outflow	Outflow
	Cameroon, U. Rep. of	0.2	0.9	−0.7	Inflow	Inflow
	China					
	Colombia	10.3	5.8	+4.5	Outflow	Outflow
	Egypt	18.8	5.5	+13.3	Outflow	Outflow
	Ethiopia	0.3	1.3	−1.0	Inflow	Inflow
	Gabon	0.1	0.3	−0.2	Inflow	Inflow
	Haiti	0.4	0.3	+0.1	Outflow	Outflow
	India	115.7	33.8	+81.9	Outflow	Outflow
	Indonesia	4.6	8.7	−4.1	Inflow	Outflow
	Iran	9.5	9.5	0.0	0	Outflow
	Jamaica	0.5	1.0	−0.5	Inflow	Inflow
	Korea, Rep. of	15.6	6.2	+9.4	Outflow	Outflow
	Lebanon	2.3	1.3	+1.0	Outflow	Outflow
	Mauritius	0.2	0.1	+0.1	Outflow	Outflow
	Nigeria	1.3	5.2	−3.9	Inflow	Inflow
	Pakistan	21.0	6.7	+14.3	Outflow	Outflow
	Philippines	14.0	5.2	+8.8	Outflow	Outflow
	Portugal	8.4	5.3	+3.1	Outflow	Outflow
	Saudi Arabia	2.6	4.3	−1.7	Inflow	Inflow
	Sri Lanka	3.2	1.5	+1.7	Outflow	Outflow
	Sudan	1.2	1.2	0.0	0	0
	Thailand	4.9	4.2	+0.7	Outflow	Outflow
	Uruguay	3.2	2.0	+1.2	Outflow	Outflow
	Yemen	0.2	0.3	−0.1	Inflow	Inflow
	Yugoslavia	21.9	10.6	+11.3	Outflow	Outflow
B. GDP $800 to $2,000	Greece	14.9	8.0	+6.9	Outflow	Outflow
	Ireland	3.6	3.3	+0.3	Outflow	Outflow
	Romania	26.9	18.4	+8.5	Outflow	Outflow
	Venezuela	10.2	5.6	+4.6	Outflow	Outflow

Table 3-16 continued

		Stock of Physicians (thousands)			Direction of Migration	
GDP Group	Country (1)	Actual (2)	Sustainable (3)	Excess (+) or Shortage (−) (2 − 3) (4)	Expected (5)	Actual (6)
C. GDP over 2,000	Australia	18.0	34.3	−16.3	Inflow	Inflow
	Austria	13.9	11.3	+2.6	Outflow	Outflow
	Canada	36.1	83.0	−46.9	Inflow	Inflow
	Germany, Fed. Rep. of	109.4	178.9	−69.5	Inflow	Inflow
	Israel	7.7	4.8	+2.9	Outflow	Inflow
	Japan	121.3	170.7	−49.4	Inflow	0
	New Zealand	3.4	5.7	−2.3	Inflow	Inflow
	Sweden	11.3	32.1	−20.8	Inflow	Inflow
	United Kingdom	74.0	103.2	−29.2	Inflow	Inflow
	United States	324.0	1023.3	−699.3	Inflow	Inflow

Source (column 2): World Health Organization, *World Health Statistics Annual 1972*, vol. 3 (Geneva: World Health Organization, 1976).

physician migration behavior was atypical, and try to find out what factors were at work there that did not apply elsewhere in the sample of countries. The atypical countries are: (1) Japan, where instead of the expected net inflow there was a net zero movement; (2) Indonesia, where although one would have expected a net inflow there was in fact a net outflow; (3) Israel, where one would have expected a net outflow but there was in fact a net inflow; and (4) Iran, where one would have expected a net zero movement but where there was instead a net outflow. In the 1970s, Iran's GDP per capita rose considerably (a four-fold increase between 1970 and 1975) and the country has until recently been experiencing an inflow of physicians.

Using these atypical countries as a starting point for the exploration of reasons why their physicians did not behave as expected, it might be suggested, for example, that the Japanese-language examination required of physicians wanting to practice in Japan acts as a deterrent to the inflow of foreign physicians. The next step would be to look at other countries that have a language that is not used elsewhere, and that nevertheless experience a net inflow, in order to see whether or not they require a language examination. (Does Ethiopia, for example, require proficiency in Amharic?) Returning to the question of Japan, it has been suggested that the cohesiveness of Japanese society would tend to be a factor militating against the outflow of physicians. [27] It would appear, however, that the outflow was negligible because Japan's supply of physicians had not reached the sustainable level, and the risk of overflow was therefore negligible.

It might be possible, through stringent and perhaps prohibitive measures, for a donor country to become a net zero-movement country even though it had a "surplus." But while such measures might temporarily solve the problem of migration, they would not necessarily solve the problem of health; and they could create even more serious problems through the resultant dissatisfaction of physicians who were obliged to remain in the country.

The message that comes across most clearly is that, in each country where the sustainable level of physician supply is not sufficient to provide adequate health care for the population as a whole, consideration should be given to ways of providing health care that are based on less expensive but nevertheless appropriate health manpower.

The Role of Expenditures in the Health Sector

The mechanism by which a country's general level of affluence conditions the sustainable level of physicians, and therefore the number of physicians who migrate, is fairly straightforward. Generally, the lower the GDP, the smaller the amount of income available for distribution to the various economic sectors, including the health sector. The smaller the amount in the health sector, the smaller the number of physicians that the country can afford to employ. The distribution of national income by economic sector is based on national priorities, and in many countries health has traditionally ranked low on the priority scale, with areas such as national defense and education taking precedence. To this can be added the fact that the distribution of GDP per inhabitant has traditionally favored the few rather than the many, with the result that large segments of the population have been deprived of the means to purchase health care, either directly or through private health-insurance schemes. This inability limits the number of physicians who have clients. Physicians who fail to achieve their professional expectations in economic and/or other terms have little choice but to seek employment in other fields in their home countries or, alternatively, to seek employment abroad in health or other fields.

From table 3-17 it can be seen that, in the richer countries, not only is total national income (GNP) high, but the proportion of that income devoted to health is also high. In the countries at the lower end of the scale of affluence, expenditure on health is, for the most part, very low both in absolute per-capita terms and as a percentage of national income: Only a very few had a health budget exceeding 1 percent of the GNP. Of the coun-

Table 3-17
Health Expenditures in Specified Countries Grouped according to GDP per Capita, circa 1971

GDP Group	*Country*	*Health Budget as Percentage of GNP (1)*	*Government Health Expenditure per Capita U.S. $ (2)*	*Physician Loss % (3)*
A. GDP less than $800	Brazil	0.2	0.80	1
	Cameroon, U.Rep. of	1.0	2.02	7
	Colombia	0.6	2.04	12
	Egypt	1.8	3.91	13
	Ethiopia	0.8	0.67	0
	Haiti	0.7	0.78	130
	India	0.9	0.91	13
	Iran	0.6	2.60	39
	Jamaica	2.7	19.54	21
	Korea, Rep. of	0.5	1.33	19
	Lebanon	0.6	3.80	41
	Philippines	0.5	1.06	67
	Sri Lanka	3.6	3.76	27
	Thailand	1.2	2.45	30
B. GDP $800 to $2,000	Romania	2.5	18.56	2
	Venezuela	4.1	43.18	3
C. GDP over $2,000	Japan	0.3	5.45	1
	United Kingdom	4.3	105.16	10

Sources (columns 1 and 2): International Bank for Development and Reconstruction, *Health: Sector Policy Paper* (Washington, D.C.: International Bank for Development and Reconstruction, 1973); (column 3): World Health Organization, *Multinational Study of the International Migration of Physicians and Nurses: Statistical Enquiry* (unpublished information).

tries in this group for which data were available, only Jamaica and Sri Lanka had devoted more than 2 percent of their GNP to health. The fact that Jamaica had a net inflow of physicians, while Sri Lanka had a net outflow, may be partly explained by Jamaica's much higher government expenditure on health per capita. Both Iran and Japan devoted a smaller-than-average proportion of GNP to the health budget. This may partly explain why, in 1970, neither of these two countries (described earlier as atypical) experienced an inflow, despite the fact that they had fewer physicians than the average for their level of GDP.

It has been postulated that there is a relationship between the migration of skilled health manpower, particularly physicians, and disparities in the allocation of health resources between the private and public sectors. With regard to those countries for which comparable data were available, the ratio of government to private expenditure on health is shown in the following table . [71]

Country	*Government/ Private-Expenditure Ratio*	*Physician Loss (Percentage)*
Jamaica	1.28	21
Korea, Rep. of	0.01	19
Sri Lanka	0.60	27
Thailand	0.12	30
Greece	0.90	11
Australia	0.36	12
Austria	1.82	15
Sweden	2.38	1
United Kingdom	15.91	10
United States	0.04	0

There appears to be no discernible relationship between physician loss and the ratio of government to private expenditure. Contrary to some of the hypotheses put forward, a study of these figures in conjunction with those in table 3-17 could lead to the conclusion that, if anything, there appears to be a greater tendency for physicians in rich countries to migrate when the health system focuses on the public sector, while in the poor countries migration appears to occur more often when the focus is on the private sector. As a corollary, one could conjecture that, in the poor countries, the total expenditure on health is so low that government expenditure either makes very little difference to the total amount of money available for health or, at the most, constitutes a small net addition to the money available. In the richer countries, government expenditure replaces private expenditure to a certain extent, as is the case in the United Kingdom. This may, in turn, have an adverse effect on the salaries of physicians.

The Role of Imbalances in Production Rates

Countries that already have more physicians than they have the economic base to employ, and that nevertheless continue to produce large numbers of the same types of manpower they are losing, risk new outflows. Conversely, countries that have fewer physicians than they can afford, and that nevertheless restrict production rates, invite further inflows.

The two-decade period 1950–1970 saw a massive expansion in the number of medical schools throughout the world, particularly in developing countries. While much of the expansion was justifiable in terms of the countries' needs, not all of it was justifiable in terms of the economic demand for physicians' services.

Table 3-18 shows the changes in the number of medical schools over the two decades in each of the forty countries of the sample. In table 3-19

Table 3-18
Increase in Number of Medical Schools between 1949 and 1970, in Countries Grouped according to GDP per Capita in 1970

		Number of Medical Schools in:		
GDP Group	*Country*	*1949 (1)*	*1966 (2)*	*1970 (3)*
A. GDP less than $800	Brazil	13	40	76
	Cameroon, U. Rep. of	0	0	1
	China (excluding Taiwan)	15	49	53
	Colombia	4	8	9
	Egypt	3	7	7
	Ethiopia	0	1	1
	Gabon	0	0	0
	Haiti	1	1	1
	India	32	86	94
	Indonesia	3	10	11
	Iran	4	7	7
	Jamaica	1	1	1
	Korea, Rep. of	6	10	14
	Lebanon	2	2	2
	Mauritius	0	0	0
	Nigeria	1	2	4
	Pakistan and Bangladesh	6	12	13
	Philippines	4	7	7
	Portugal	3	3	3
	Saudi Arabia	0	0	1
	Sri Lanka	1	2	2
	Sudan	1	1	1
	Thailand	2	3	4
	Uruguay	1	1	1
	Yemen	0	0	0
	Yugoslavia	6	9	9

Table 3-18 continued

GDP Group	*Country*	*Number of Medical Schools in:* 1949 (1)	1966 (2)	1970 (3)
B. GDP $800 to $2,000	Greece	2	2	2
	Ireland	4	4	4
	Romania	5	5	6
	Venezuela	3	7	7
C. GDP over $2,000	Australia	4	8	8
	Austria	3	3	3
	Canada	11	13	16
	Germany, Fed. Rep. of	19	22	27
	Israel	1	2	3
	Japan	44	46	50
	New Zealand	1	1	2
	Sweden	4	5	6
	United Kingdom	28	28	30
	United States	84	96	116

Source: World Health Organization, *World Directory of Medical Schools 1970* (Geneva: World Health Organization, 1973).

this growth in medical schools, along with the average annual production of physicians relative to stock, is compared with each country's position relative to the sustainable level of physician coverage. The countries are grouped according to the migration behavior of physicians. Rationally, one would expect low production rates in countries that had an excess of physicians and had lost a portion of them through migration, and higher production rates in countries that had fewer physicians than the sustainable number and had experienced physician inflows. In fact, the opposite situation obtained. The highest production rates existed in those countries that were already saturated with physicians and experiencing an overflow; the median production rate for this group was 6 percent. With normal attrition at about 3 percent per annum, this was about double the natural replacement rate. In the low-movement countries the median production rate was 5 percent and in the recipient countries 4 percent, scarcely higher than the natural attrition rate. The following discussion focuses on the recipient countries, the low-movement countries, and the donor countries, in that order. It is followed in turn by a discussion of physician production in Latin America, based on a special case study of that region.[1]

Table 3-19
Production of Physicians and Migration Behavior

Country	New Medical Schools Opened 1950–1970 (1)	Annual Production of Physicians as Percentage of Stock (2)	Excess or Shortage of Physicians per 10,000 Population (3)
Donor Countries			
Austria	0	4	+1.6
Colombia	5	5	+2.0
Egypt	4	8	+3.9
Greece	0	6	+7.7
Haiti	0	15	+0.1
India	62	7	+1.5
Iran	3	8	0.0
Ireland	0	12	+0.8
Korea, Rep. of	8	4	+2.9
Lebanon	0	4	+3.7
Pakistan and Bangladesh	7	6	+2.7
Philippines	3	8	+2.2
Sri Lanka	1	5	+1.3
Thailand	2	6	+0.1
Yugoslavia	3	8	+5.4
Low net-movement countries			
Brazil	63	6	+1.4
Germany, Fed. Rep. of	8	4	−11.3
Indonesia	8	13	−0.4
Japan	6	3	−4.7
Portugal	0	4	+3.5
Romania	1	5	+4.1
Sudan	0	6	0.0
Uruguay	0	7	+3.7
Venezuela	4	6	+0.7
Recipient countries			
Australia	4	5	−12.7
Canada	5	3	−21.5
Ethiopia	1	6	−0.4
Israel	2	2	+9.6
Jamaica	0	4	−2.7
New Zealand	1	3	−7.8
Nigeria	4	6	−0.7
Sweden	2	5	−26.2
United Kingdom	2	4	−5.2
United States	32	3	−33.2

Sources (column 1): Table 3-18; (column 2): World Health Organization, *Multinational Study of the International Migration of Physicians and Nurses: Statistical Enquiry* (unpublished information); (column 3): Table 3-15.

Notes: Data in column 2 represent average annual production of new graduates relative to domestic stock for the years 1960–1973. The number of years for which data on production were available varied from country to country. In the case of Ethiopia, Indonesia, Republic of Korea, Lebanon, and the United Kingdom, information was available only for the year 1970. Countries with no graduates in 1970 are excluded.

The *recipient countries,* as always, fall into two categories: developing and developed. Among the developing recipient countries, most have not yet become self-sufficient with regard to physician production, although Nigeria is planning such a large expansion of physician production (five medical schools are planned, in addition to the five existing in 1970) that it risks over shooting its sustainable level. [11] The developed-country recipients (plus Jamaica) all have rather low production rates. It would almost seem that they are content to import their physicians while producing very few at home. The situation in Israel is perhaps a special case in that the immigration of physicians is only part of a wider immigration movement, but even in Israel the age structure of its physician population is top-heavy. [37]

Among the *low-movement countries,* Indonesia had a slight physician shortage and a very high production rate; it remains to be seen whether this will push Indonesia over the brink to join the ranks of the heavy-donor countries. Portugal appeared to be pursuing a rational policy with respect to production. The Federal Republic of Germany is a special case in that it is a donor of medical education; about 10 percent of its medical-school enrollment in the early 1970s consisted of foreign students. This means that its effectve production rate has been approximately 3 percent, or somewhat lower than that needed to stem the inflow resulting from its physician shortage vis à vis the sustainable level. Brazil experienced an enormous increase in the number of its medical schools but, in recent years the increased output of these schools is not apparent from the production rates shown in table 3-19, which are based on historical data.

Among the *donor countries,* only Iran appears not to have had an excess of physicians, not so much because of low production rates but because about one-third of the graduates each year had migrated. Iran's rapid economic expansion in recent years probably increased its capacity to retain its graduates; for a while, in fact, Iran appeared to be on its way to becoming a recipient country. The only donor country that seemed to be following a rational policy with respect to production was Austria, which had an excess of physicians, had not increased the number of medical schools, and had maintained a fairly low rate of production in relation to stock. All the others appeared to be desperately trying to compensate for the outflow in what was, effectively, the most uneconomical manner possible. It should be noted that, while Ireland's production rate appears enormous, the figures are somewhat misleading in that a large proportion of the medical graduates are foreign. In 1970 foreigners constituted 42 percent of the graduates. If this proportion were deducted from the 12 percent production rate recorded in table 3-19, the average annual production rate could be considered as 7 percent, which is still somewhat high but not so startling.

Because Latin America's migrant physicians have generally gone to the

United States rather than to other countries, it may be interesting to note the situation in that region with regard to the production of physicians. Table 3-20 shows that medical-education facilities and enrollment have been expanding rapidly in a number of countries. Whereas in 1967-1968 there were 100 medical schools in Central and South America, by 1971-1972 there were 158, representing an increase of 58 percent. During the same period, Brazil alone opened 42 new medical schools, making a total of 73 for Brazil in 1971-1972. More recent but unpublished information suggests that there are at least 45 more medical schools in the region than were officially reported for 1971-1972 (3 more in Brazil, 5 more in Colombia, and 37 more in Mexico, or totals of 76, 14, and 62 in the three countries, respectively). This would bring the overall total of medical schools for the region up to 203, double the number officially reported as existing in 1967-1968. Between the years 1967-1968 and 1975-1976, the number in Brazil more than doubled, that in Colombia doubled, and that in Mexico trebled.

The number of students enrolled in the region's medical schools increased from 98,245 in 1967-1968 to 159,759 in 1971-1972, an increase of 63 percent (table 3-20). In the four-year period, the number enrolled in Bra-

Table 3-20
Expansion of Medical Schools and Medical-Student Enrollment in Central and South America between the Academic Years 1967-1968 and 1971-1972

	Schools		*Students Enrolled*		
Country	*Number in 1967-1968*	*Number in 1971-1972*	*Number in 1967-1968*	*Number in 1971-1972*	*Percentage Increase*
Brazil	31	73	21,907	44,074	102
Mexico	21	25	20,127	41,675	107
Argentina	9	9	27,790	29,891	8
Colombia	7	9	3,572	4,547	27
Venezuela	6	7	5,491	6,232	13
Peru	4	6	2,580	3,487	35
Bolivia	3	3	2,179	1,788[a]	—
Chile	3	5	2,320	2,546	10
Ecuador	3	5	1,660	4,638	179
Dominican Republic	1	2	1,109	4,087	268
Cuba	2	3	4,516	7,098	57
Other	11	11	4,994	9,686	94
Total	100	158	98,245	159,749	63

Source: M.I. Rodriguez, "El estudiante de medecina—su distribución en las Américas, 1971-1972. *Educacioń Medica y Salud* 8(1974):360-389.

[a]Refers to only two schools.

zil increased by over 22,000 (102 percent increase) and that in Mexico by over 21,000 (107 percent increase). The expansion of enrollment in Mexico is partly due to the larger number of students from the United States who were studying there in the early 1970s. With the current expansion of places in schools in the United States, and the special efforts being made to accommodate American citizens who have had at least two years of training abroad, the number of Americans studying in Mexico is expected to decline.

While the overall percentage increase in enrollment in Argentina is rather small for the four-year period considered, it has been reported that in the past few years at least one medical school (Faculty of Medicine, University of Buenos Aires) has greatly liberalized its admission policy. [18] As a result, first-year admissions to the school increased from 2,433 in 1973 to 12,499 in 1974, an increase of over 10,000 or 414 percent in a single year. Stated otherwise, in 1974 there were *five* times as many first-year admissions as in the preceding year, and *thirteen* times as many as in 1969. This massive increase is more than anything a response to the large-scale demand for medical education as a part of the growing demand for university education in all fields—a demand not limited to Argentina alone. As can be seen in table 3-20, medical school enrollment has increased considerably in most countries of the region. This demand does not appear to be related to demand for services. Moreover, without the necessary increase in institutions and equipment (as in Argentina, for example, where there was no increase in the number of medical schools), the results are crowding, lower quality of teaching, inadequate learning, poor student evaluation, and so on. The products of such a system may find it difficult to obtain employment in the country, particularly if the supply of physicians outstrips the demand. Emigration may be the only solution for many such graduates.

It is too early to measure the full impact that the 63 percent increase in enrollment in the region may have with regard to emigration from the region, although the numbers of graduates from Latin American medical schools found in the United States in 1974 reflect notable increases over the numbers found there in 1970—242 more from Brazil, 299 more from Colombia, and 735 more from Mexico, for example. The higher number from Mexico may be partly the result of the higher number of U.S. nationals returning home after graduation in Mexico. While there have been increases from the three countries in which medical school expansion was the greatest, the increases were not as large as might be expected. The probable explanation is that, because medical education takes six years in Brazil and Mexico, and seven years in Colombia, a number of students are not counted in the migration data for 1974. In the case of Brazil, another possible explanation is that the rapid rate of growth in GNP per capita (6 percent per year over the period 1965–1973) has increased the opportunities for employment.

An interesting point that emerged from one study of Latin American schools is that countries that have been reluctant to expand medical education have ended up by seeing large numbers of their nationals going abroad for study. [42] If these students were to return home after graduation they could well defeat the purpose of national policy. The main conclusion to be drawn is that the demand for medical education seems to be totally unrelated to employment opportunities in the home country (let alone to the actual need for medical manpower) and to be irrepressible. For those countries that are trying to plan their future supply of physicians, if they are not to end up by producing physicians for the export market, it is imperative that they bear in mind the numbers they can afford to employ—their sustainable level. Thus, for example, a level of eight physicians per 10,000 population (the target set for the year 1980 according to the Ten Year Plan for the Americas) would be well above the level sustainable by most countries in the region. Even on the assumption that real per-capita GDP will double by the year 2000, fewer than half the countries in the region would be able to afford at least eight physicians per 10,000 population (Argentina, Brazil, Barbados, Chile, Costa Rica, Jamaica, Mexico, Panama, Trinidad and Tobago, Uruguay, and Venezuela).

The lesson to be drawn from this analysis is that, if the emigration of physicians can be attributed in part to an excess of physicians in relation to effective economic demand for their services, then it would seem to be unrealistic to pour more money into expanding the supply of physicians. Apart from (and perhaps in spite of) revolutions, effective economic demand for physician services can grow only to the extent that GDP grows *and* is more evenly distributed, and even then it may take some time before the sustainable level of physician stock in some countries catches up with the actual level. Under such circumstances there should be, if anything, a cutback in production rates, accompanied by increased production of health manpower who are less costly to train and maintain but who are, nevertheless, appropriate for the tasks to be performed. While it seems clear that countries with more physicians than the sustainable level should not increase production, it does not automatically follow that cutting back production will cause the emigration rate to fall. This point is clearly observed in the case of the Philippines, where a cut in the production rate was followed by a fall in the physician/population ratio, rather than by a slowing down of emigration. It would seem that the rate of outflow is not sensitive to decreases in production while there is an excess of 2.2 physicians per 10,000 population. Moreover, physician supply is not automatically reduced by a cutback in local production, given that the demand for medical education is so great in many countries that students failing to obtain admission to medical schools in their home countries will go abroad to obtain it. This was shown to be the case in a number of Latin American countries, and may well be so elsewhere. If a sizable proportion of those who study abroad return to their homelands after graduation, the supply of physicians will increase despite restrictions on the domestic production of physicians.

As noted earlier in this section, the increasing demand for medical education is part of the tremendous upsurge in demand for higher education. In many countries, the education sector has developed much faster than the health sector. In the Philippines, for example, government expenditure for education accounted for 13 percent of the national budget in 1974, compared to only 3 percent for health. It might be added that the demand for higher education, like that for medical education, appears to be completely unrelated to employment opportunities.

The Role of Irrelevant Education and Training

Perhaps the most universally accepted explanation of why professional health workers, particularly physicians, migrate is that the education and training they receive have little relevance to the type of health services and care needed by the majority of people in the countries from which they migrate. In most countries of the world, donor and recipient alike, the training of health workers (in terms of curriculum content and the methods, equipment, and facilities used in the teaching and learning process) is essentially geared toward meeting the world economic demand for personal health care, as opposed to the more pervasive needs of the majority of the population. The problem is aggravated by the fact that the effective economic demand for the type of health care implicit in the training provided is far greater in affluent recipient countries than in poor donor countries, where the disease patterns are essentially different from those in the affluent recipient countries and where only a small segment of the population can afford the types of health care implicit in the training provided to professional health workers.

Physicians trained according to developed-country standards are thus not only unable to function efficiently in developing countries but are so expensive to train, and subsequently to pay, that most developing countries cannot possibly meet their basic health-service needs by using this type of manpower. Considering the ramifications of the problem of irrelevant education, and the lack of readily available information on the various pertinent subfactors, the problem and its possible relation to migration can be assessed realistically only within and by the countries themselves, since each country's situation is unique. The following sections contain several findings pertinent to the problem of irrelevant education and training, which point to some of the areas that require on-the-spot investigation in order to determine the impact of irrelevant education and training on migration and, in particular, on health.

Specialization. As far as intercountry comparisons are concerned, the only evidence available that might shed some light on the relationship between migration and irrelevant education is that provided by a study carried out in the United States in 1970. [35] The specific subfactor concerned was the degree of specialization among physicians in a sample of thirty-two countries. Table 3-21 presents the relevant data from that study. If the high proportions of specialists in Colombia and Peru are representative of those for other countries of Latin America, then at least two out of every three physicians in the region are specialists. The proportions of specialists among physicians in the Asian countries vary greatly, from 4 percent in Pakistan to 75 and 80 percent in Thailand and Sri Lanka, respectively. The proportions in the European countries are relatively low, ranging from 30 to 40 percent. In essence, the finding was that there is a highly significant and positive relationship between physician migration to the United States and the proportion of specialists among physicians in the donor countries. The study concludes that, where the proportion is relatively high, the medical profession is much more like that of the United States, which encourages specialization; where it is low, the physician's teachers (and role models) are likely to emphasize general practice, in which case the physician would be less attracted to American-style medicine. Another conclusion is that a high concentration of specialists in countries where the effective market demand for them is low makes it very difficult for new entrants to the profession to obtain a reasonable income, and thus makes them more likely to migrate.

A study cited earlier, concerning candidates for the ECFMG examination in the United States, showed that over half the candidates claimed to have had specialty training before leaving their countries. [31]

Health Research. The orientation of a country's medical-education program can hardly be disassociated from the orientation of its health-research program. The orientation of health research, in turn, can hardly be disassociated from, among other things, the manner in which the research is funded, the particular interests of the sponsoring agency, and the particular interests of the investigators. Some interesting observations in this area appear in the report of a study carried out by the Pan American Health Organization on health research in Latin America. [40]

According to that report, the health-research program in Latin America had until recently been supported largely by governments and foundations outside Latin America. While acknowledging the undeniable value of such support, the report also points to its important adverse consequences.

1. Imposition of inappropriate models: This often occurs when students returning from study abroad bring back with them not only skills but also values that are inappropriate in their home countries; dependence on foreign funds has fostered the tendency to look abroad for guidance in such matters as institutional governance and administration, research planning, and patterns of graduate education.
2. Inappropriate transfer of responsibility: When too much money for biomedical research is received from outside a country, a government may tend to ignore its responsibility to finance biomedical research;
3. Establishment of inappropriate research priorities: While external funds may amount to only 10 to 15 percent of total research costs (usually for such things as laboratory supplies, equipment, research animals, and technicians), the nature of these supplies and the person responsible for directing how this relatively small sum is spent can determine the course of research. This is how a small external investment has, in the past, exercised a strong influence over large segments of the health-research program of a nation. Most of the research funds supplied by the government of the United States (rather than by foundations) have been directed, not toward the development of science in Latin America or toward problems important to the region, but instead toward the financing of research relevant to the tasks of various parts of the U.S. government. For example, grants and contracts were awarded almost entirely for sophisticated laboratory research, and grants were often awarded to the individual investigator without reference to university or national authorities, in which case the priority-setting factor was the special interest of the investigator.

The Role of Imbalances in the Health Team

As indicated previously, countries that lose physicians because they are producing too many are likely to be those suffering from a general imbalance in their education systems that results in a shortage of middle-level manpower in relation to numbers of university graduates. With respect to physicians, this factor manifests itself in a shortage of support staff such as nurses and other nursing personnel. Moreover, it has been suggested that, because physicians have been traditionally trained in a way that leads them to expect support from a team of other health workers, they are likely to find it difficult to function in situations where such support is lacking in quantity or quality, and thus are likely to seek work where an adequate team will be assured.

Table 3-22 shows, for the countries in the sample, the number of professional nurses, as well as the number of nursing personnel as a whole, per

Table 3-21
Percentage of Specialists among Physicians in Specified Countries

Country	*Year*	*Percentage of Specialists*
Colombia	1965	73
Peru	1964	67
Afghanistan	1968	62
Indonesia	1968	11
Iran	1964	21
Korea, Rep. of	1968	14
Malaysia	1968	40
Nepal	1965	16
Pakistan	1964	4
Singapore	1968	53
Sri Lanka	1968	80
Thailand	1968	74
Turkey	1964	74
Vietnam	1968	17
Denmark	1964	32
France	1964	33
Germany, Fed. Rep. of	1964	40
Norway	1964	41
United Kingdom	1964	41
Australia	1968	53
New Zealand	1968	58
Netherlands	1964	34
Sweden	1964	39
Canada	1963	49
Puerto Rico	1964	39
United States	1963	62

Source: H. Luft, *Determinants of the Flow of Physicians to the United States* (Santa Monica, Calif.: Rand Corporation, 1970).

Note: The source did not indicate whether the percentages referred to those *trained* in a specialty or to those who reported that their *work* was primarily in a specialty field. In the case of Colombia, for example, only 34.3 percent of physicians were found by R. Paredes Manrique and C. Agualimpia, *Study of Human Resources for Health and Medical Education in Colombia: Methods and Results* (Bogota: Ministry of Public Health and Colombian Association of Medical Faculties, 1972), to have been certified as specialists by the Colombian Association of Medical Faculties, in 1968.

physician. Within each GDP group the countries are ranked according to physician-migration behavior (from high gain to high loss). The data presented in table 3-22 show that the health-team ratios differed markedly between the upper and lower halves of the list of countries in each GDP

Table 3-22
Number of Nurses and Nursing Personnel per Physician, in Countries Grouped by GDP per Capita [1970] and Ranked according to Percentage Gains and Losses through Physician Migration

GDP Group	*Country*	*Percentage Net Gain (+) or Loss (−) of Physicians (1)*	*Nurses per Physician (2)*	*Nursing Personnel per Physician (3)*[a]
A. GDP less than $800	Ethiopia	+95	2.4	3.1
	Gabon	+80	2.7	9.6
	Cameroon, U. Rep. of	+63	5.2	11.6
	Saudi Arabia	+44	1.1	1.1
	Yemen	+40	1.1	2.4
	Jamaica	+9	3.7	4.5
	Nigeria	+6	6.8	7.3
	Sudan	0	8.0	10.1
	Brazil	−1	0.4	0.4
	Portugal	−2	0.5	1.1
	Uruguay	−3	0.2	0.2
	Indonesia	−3	3.4	5.3
	Yugoslavia	−7	1.5	2.0
	Colombia	−8	0.3	1.5
	Pakistan and Bangladesh	−12	0.3	0.4
	India	−13	0.7	1.1
	Egypt	−13	0.3	2.1
	Korea, Rep. of	−19	1.2	1.6
	Thailand	−26	1.2	2.6
	Sri Lanka	−27	2.0	3.1
	Lebanon	−33	0.7	1.4
	Iran	−38	0.4	1.7
	Philippines	−67	0.6	1.5
	Mauritius	−72	4.8	8.3
	Haiti	−130	1.0	1.4
B. GDP $800 to $2,000	Romania	−2	1.3	1.8
	Venezuela	−3	0.7	2.3
	Greece	−11	0.4	0.5
	Ireland	−121	5.4	5.4

[a]Figures represent all those categories of nursing personnel (including professional nurses) used in World Health Organization, *World Health Statistics Annual, 1973* (Geneva: World Health Organization, 1973) to determine the ratio of nursing and midwifery personnel to population.

Table 3-22 continued

GDP Group	*Country*	*Percentage Net Gain (+) or Loss (−) of Physicians (1)*	*Nurses per Physician (2)*	*Nursing Personnel per Physician (3)*
C. GDP over $2,000	United States	+21	2.4	4.0
	United Kingdom	+15	2.0	3.0
	Israel	+20	0.6	
	Canada	+13	3.3	4.7
	Australia	+12	3.1	
	New Zealand	+5	5.2	5.6
	Sweden	+4	3.1	4.7
	Germany, Fed. Rep. of	+1	1.2	1.5
	Japan	−0	1.3	2.8
	Austria	−10	1.1	1.6

Sources: World Health Organization, *Multinational Study of the International Migration of Physicians and Nurses: Statistical Enquiry* (unpublished information); and World Health Organization, *World Health Statistics Annual, 1973* (Geneva: World Health Organization, 1973).

Table 3-23
Weighted Averages of Health-Team Ratios for Upper and Lower Halves of Each GDP Group

GDP Group	*Weighted Average of the Number, per Physician, of:* Nurses	*All Nursing Personnel*	*Percentage Loss or Gain*
Group A			
Top 13 countries	1.1	1.4	+95 to −7
Bottom 12 countries	0.6	1.2	−9 to −130
Group B			
Top 2 countries	1.1	2.0	−2 to −3
Bottom 2 countries	1.3	1.5	−11 to −121
Group C			
Top 5 countries	2.5	3.9	+21 to +12
Bottom 5 countries	1.4	2.4	+5 to −10

group. The weighted averages for the upper and lower halves of each GDP group, together with the percentage net gains or losses in physician stock, are presented in table 3-23.

Group B in table 3-23 is too small to provide any valid conclusion, but in both group A and group B there would seem to be significantly more professional nurses and nursing personnel as a whole among the top group of countries than among the bottom. For group A this means that, in countries experiencing a net gain or a low loss, the average number of nurses per physician was 1.1, while for countries with a net loss of over 8 percent there was, on average, only 1 nurse to nearly 2 physicians. The equivalent ratios for nursing personnel as a whole were 1.4 for countries experiencing a net gain or a low loss, and 1.2 for those with a net loss of over 8 percent. In group C, also, those countries experiencing a high net gain of physicians had more nurses and total nursing personnel per physician than did those countries experiencing a smaller gain or a loss.

The Role of Income Differentials

The differences between donor and recipient countries with regard to the income of physicians has often been cited as a factor in migration. Reference has often been made to the difference between the income of physicians in the United States and in some of the major donor countries. Various studies of the motives of migrants show that individual migrants often indicate income differentials as a reason for migrating. While this may be the immediate reason, there is no evidence to show that income differentials alone, without other factors such as employment opportunities, are a basic cause of migration.

For migrant physicians, income differentials obviously determine the direction of their migration, in that they tend to move to countries where the average income of physicians is higher than is the case in their homelands. However, not all countries where the average income of physicians is low relative to that in the major recipient countries experience migration losses.

In countries where physician incomes are low because expenditure on health is low and physician supply is high relative to the amount of money available to pay them, emigration does take place. Under such circumstances, low incomes constitute a symptom of imbalances in the employment market rather than a factor directly responsible for migration.

In donor countries, physician income can be measured in one of two ways: (1) relative to incomes in potential recipient countries such as the United States, in which case it becomes a truism to speak of income differentials, given that incomes in the major recipient countries are the highest in the world; and (2) relative to other incomes in the same country.

The little information that exists shows that, if the income of physicians in a country is compared to the nation's per-capita income, then physicians in the major donor countries usually earn relatively more than their colleagues in the receiving countries. This is illustrated in table 3-24, which shows, for sixteen of the forty countries in the sample, the relationship

Table 3-24
Relationship between the Annual Average Income of Physicians and the per Capita Income of the Population in Specified Countries, 1968

Country	*Per Capita Income (U.S. $) (1)*	*Physician Income (U.S. $) (2)*	*Ratio of Physician Income to per Capita Income (2 ÷ 1) (3)*
India	73	562	7.7
Indonesia	86	190	2.2
Pakistan	112	1,340	12.0
Thailand	127	4,433	34.9
Sri Lanka	133	5,530	41.6
Rep. of Korea	159	1,208	7.6
Philippines	233	3,939	16.9
Iran	252	4,134	16.4
Colombia	273	5,250	19.2
United Kingdom	1,437	9,600	6.7
Germany, Fed. Rep. of	1,670	12,807	7.7
New Zealand	1,714	11,943	7.0
Australia	1,788	12,159	6.8
Canada	2,254	24,477	10.9
Sweden	2,821	14,299	5.1
United States of America	3,551	30,060	8.5

Source: H. Luft, *Determinants of the Flow of Physicians to the United States* (Santa Monica, Calif.: Rand Corporation, 1970).

Note: Conversion from local currency to U.S. $ is based on rates for 1969.

between the average annual income of physicians in 1968 and the average income of the population for the same year. It would appear that the income of a physician in the donor countries as a group was about 18 times higher than the average per-capita income of the population (the range being from 2.2 to 41.6 times higher), while in the receiving countries it was about 8 times higher (the range being from 5.1 to 10.9 times higher). This would suggest that the income of physicians in most of the donor countries is more than the population can afford to pay on any large scale and that, therefore, the risk of physician unemployment and eventual migration is great.

Since very little information was available as to the proportion of the physicians who emigrated that had been unemployed or underemployed in their homelands, it was not possible to gauge the extent to which the factor of employment played a role in decisions to migrate. There are indications, however, that a large proportion of the younger physicians moving to the United States make the decision to migrate while still at medical school or soon after graduation. [47] Whether this is related to their perceived lack of employment opportunities at home is not known, but would be an essential area of study in countries wishing to regulate migration.

In Indonesia, where the income of a physician in 1968 was only about twice as high as the per-capita income of the population, the net loss of physicians through migration was only 3 percent, as compared with the much higher losses in those donor countries where the income of a physician was many times higher than that of the population per capita. Indonesia is also the only one of the developing countries listed in table 3-24 that had a shortage of physicians relative to what its economic base could afford. In other words, presumably Indonesia could afford to employ the physicians it had and, therefore, few physicians left the country despite the fact that their earnings were not much higher than those of the general population.

For countries where the per-capita income of physicians is between 10 and 40 times higher than that of the population generally (and much higher when compared with that of the masses in the lowest-income group), it becomes obvious that increasing the income of physicians as an incentive to keep them in the country would only widen the gap between their income and that of the poor, and thus reduce the effective economic demand for medical care. To increase the rate of production of physicians under such circumstances would compound the problem, and would only lead to further migration.

The Role of Language

While the teaching of medicine in a language other than that commonly spoken in a country is often cited as a factor causing migration, the WHO multinational study found no evidence to support this theory. On the other hand, the teaching of medicine in a foreign language can be viewed as a facilitating factor, conditioning the directions of the migratory flows. The findings of the WHO study in this regard can be summarized as follows:

Link Language	*Actual Percentage*	*Expected Percentage*
English	95	92
French	27	9
English/French	100	92
German	11	5
Arabic	35	2
Other	5	1

The first column shows, for each group of physicians who came from countries having a common language of instruction, the percentage who went to countries where the particular language indicated is spoken. The second column shows the percentage that would have obtained had there been no language links. Thus, for example, the first row of the table indicates that of all physicians who migrated from countries where the language of instruction is English, 95 percent went to countries where English is a national language; had there been no language link, the percentage might have been about 92 percent. The conclusion to be drawn is that rather strong links exist between the language of tuition in medical schools and the direction of physician migration.

The fact that roughly half the FMGs in the United States come from countries where English is neither the national nor the teaching language suggests that, while language may be one factor conditioning the direction of migration, it is not the only one. For example, the flow of physicians from Central and South America to the United States (rather than elsewhere) is probably due to the geographic proximity of the two areas, aside from the sheer strength of the pull factors in the United States.

Political Crises and Migration

A certain amount of migration results from the sudden reordering of societies. This type of migration is likely to be sudden, to reach a high peak within a short period of time, and to decline almost as rapidly. The effect of such sudden crises on physician migration from Cuba, Czechoslovakia, and Hungary has been noted. A study of the brain drain from Argentina to the United States during the period 1950–1970 showed a significant correlation between political crises in Argentina and peaks of physician emigration. [39]

While the cause of migration in such instances might be seen as lying outside the health sector, it is difficult to define the boundary, given that a profound political shift is also likely to affect the health sector and the conditions of workers in that sector. The Cuban revolution, for example, caused a profound political change in the country, followed a year or two later by a complete reorganization of the health sector. It is impossible to ascertain which of the two factors, the political changes as such or the changes in the health sector as a particular but less sudden part of the political changes, played a greater role in the exodus of physicians that depleted the domestic stock by over 1,000 between 1961 and 1962. Physicians appear to migrate in response to some types of political shifts and not to others. For example, there appears to have been no such response to political upheavals in Brazil in 1964 or in Indonesia in 1968. Clearly, physicians do not migrate when the political shift is likely to enhance, or at least not diminish, their interests.

Legislation and Migration

Aside from the numerous factors that cause health manpower to feel the need to migrate, other factors have facilitated the movement of many. Among these, the two main ones are (1) the relative ease with which foreign health manpower has been able (at least within the past ten years) to obtain permission to practice in some countries, despite what appear to be relatively rigid controls on the practice of medicine, and (2) the relatively permissive policies of the major recipient countries with regard to the immigration of highly skilled and trained manpower.

The record shows that migration policies and practices in highly developed countries have nearly always been more influential in determining the pattern of migration than have those in developing countries. This notion is clearly demonstrated by the results of the United States' unilateral decision, in 1965, to lower the quota for immigration generally from the Western Hemisphere and raise it for highly skilled manpower from other parts of the world. It is also demonstrated by the relatively heavy inflow of foreign physicians into Canada, the Federal Republic of Germany, and the United Kingdom, which also around that time started to relax their restrictions on the employment of highly skilled foreign health manpower, although recently all four countries have been trying to reverse this policy.

It is presumed that each country has regulations, explicit or implicit, governing the practice of medicine by health manpower born and/or trained outside the country. A WHO publication entitled *Equivalence of Medical Qualifications: a Survey of Existing Legislation* contains details of the regulations existing in 1967 in forty-two countries, of which eighteen happen to be countries included in the forty used as the sample for the WHO multinational study of health-manpower migration. [67]

From an analysis of the various regulations pertaining to medical practice, one gains the impression that, in general, physicians trained in one country would have considerable difficulty in obtaining permission to practice in another. If the provisions are to be interpreted strictly and literally, it would appear that there is no such thing as *automatic* equivalence and international recognition of qualifications. In some countries, such as Canada and the United States, both of which have a federal system of government, equivalence does not exist even within the country itself. Thus, a physician who qualifies in a particular province of Canada is not automatically entitled to practice in another province; nor is a physician who qualifies in a particular state in the United States entitled automatically to practice in another state.

It is only rarely that a country's legislation contains provisions as to the equivalence and validation of *incomplete* studies effected abroad, by either national or foreign students who wish to continue their studies in the country concerned. Among the forty-two countries dealt with in the WHO survey, only Belgium, France, and the Federal Republic of Germany had such provisions in 1967. On the other hand, most countries surveyed had provisions concerning the validation of diplomas in medicine obtained abroad. In this respect, the provisions may be divided roughly into two groups: those that permit the recognition of foreign qualifications only in exceptional cases, and those that make such recognition subject to certain conditions, the latter varying from country to country with regard to the degree of flexibility.

Because of the marked differences in the provisions, and the lack of information as to *how* (and even, in some instances, *whether*) the provisions are applied, generalization is difficult. In some instances, moreover, the provisions are so worded that they can be interpreted in the manner considered most feasible at any particular time by those responsible for deciding which, and how many, physicians born and/or trained elsewhere will be allowed to practice in the country concerned. Essentially, the supply/demand market determines how provisions are interpreted and applied. Furthermore, no legislation is binding for all time; as stated earlier, some of the major recipient countries are changing their regulations in order to respond to new requirements. Such changes are likely to affect the pattern of physician migration throughout the world. The appendix provides details on migration legislation and licensing practices as they pertain to the foreign medical graduate in the United States.

Note

1. The case study on Latin America was specially requested by the Fogarty International Center (US/DHEW/NIH). It was carried out at WHO Headquarters, Geneva, and was based on material compiled in connection with the WHO Multinational Study of the International Migration of Physicians and Nurses. The case study is in the process of publication by the center as part of its anthology, "Biomedical Research Trends in Latin America and the Caribbean."

4 Consequences of Migration

The literature on migration contains a variety of views on the consequences of physician migration. Statistical evidence of the loss to the donor countries, and the gain to the recipient countries, of the cost of educating those physicians who migrated, is as contradictory as it is abundant. The extent of the loss or gain is not clear, given the diverse and often unquantifiable variables that need to be considered. Lack of information has also made it impossible to determine the extent to which the donor countries are compensated for their losses through foreign aid and through remittances sent by the migrants to their relatives at home.

Much has also been said about the impact of physician migration on the status of health care in donor and recipient countries alike. However, the methods used to measure this are so indirect as to be almost useless. The most that can be shown is that in the receiving country (in this case the United States), more people may be receiving care than if the immigration had not taken place. Given the heavy concentration of foreign physicians in urban areas and in hospitals in the United States, it is doubtful whether formerly deprived segments of the population outside these areas are being better served as a result of the inflow of foreign physicians. It is also not clear whether more people in the donor countries would be receiving care if emigration had not taken place, since no information is available on the number of migrants who were employed or employable in their home countries prior to their emigration. Given the relatively low economic capacity of many of the donor countries, it is unlikely that many more people could afford to avail themselves of the services of these health workers if they remained.

In any case, the migration of health manpower cannot help the efforts of those who are responsible for planning health services and health manpower. If the aim is to increase the coverage of health services, then a continuous drain of skilled personnel is a serious problem. In the recipient countries, the inflow of foreign health manpower obviates the need for structural changes in the health system. This, too, can have serious implications in the long run.

Opposing Views

The debate over the consequences of health-manpower migration is no less vehement than the debate over the determinants of that migration. The line is clearly drawn between two opposing forces. On the one hand are those who view the migration phenomenon from the *international* perspective, and who claim that the donor countries produce more highly skilled manpower, particularly physicians, than they can economically absorb; that those who cannot be absorbed migrate; and that, through their migration and gainful employment elsewhere, the total world output is raised, thereby benefiting mankind as a whole. To enhance this argument, they also point to the worldwide contributions made by individual migrants through their research activities outside their native lands (for example, Waksman, a native of the USSR, discovered streptomycin through work in the United States; and Florey, a native of Australia, contributed to the development of penicillin through work in the United Kingdom). They further argue that, with respect to the donor countries: (1) they are not really losing, given that they had been unable to use effectively the skills of those who migrated; (2) their losses are offset by foreign aid, by the remittances of the emigrants, and by the goodwill created abroad by the emigrants; and (3) they are able to stockpile intellectual resources abroad until some future time when these can be repatriated and effectively used at home.

It would appear, however, that statements defending migration were more frequent a decade ago than they are today, and that current value judgments on the migration of high-level personnel, even in recipient countries, would be less favorable.

These arguments have been countered by those who believe that the migration of skilled personnel represents less a gain to the world than a loss to individual nations. Some of the counterarguments follow.

1. While there is no denying the special contributions to mankind as a whole made by such migrants as Waksman and Florey, the same does not apply to the many thousands of other highly trained health manpower who migrate, and whose work abroad can in no way be construed as being of benefit to the donor countries. Moreover, given the tremendous existing disparities within and between countries with regard to the health and welfare of various segments of the population, the world cannot be considered as a single aggregate for the purpose of rationalizing a phenomenon that leads to further disparities.

2. The cost of training high-level health manpower involves not only material resources but also time. It is essentially a social cost that must be repaid, in one form or another, to the society that bears the cost.

3. In assessing the determinants and consequences of migration, those who advocate, or at least try to defend, the free flow of human capital often

fail to distinguish between professional manpower and less highly trained workers or skilled laborers. The determinants and, perhaps even more markedly, the consequences of the migration of the latter groups may be entirely different from those pertaining to professional manpower, if for no other reason than that they represent a smaller investment and a generally more ample supply. Furthermore, such advocates often fail to distinguish between the different categories of professional manpower yet the determinants and consequences of the migration of physicians, for example, may be entirely different from those pertaining to nuclear scientists and engineers. The mere fact that physicians essentially provide services directly to people, and that population size has always been a factor in determining the need for physicians, places such manpower in a category that is very different from that of manpower who are involved in the development of products or production processes, or in the production of goods. In more practical terms, the argument would be that, when even one physician emigrates, hundreds of people in his homeland may actually or potentially be denied health care. Only in exceptional cases, such as those of Florey and Waksman, would people in the donor country stand to benefit. A further argument along this line is that a large part of whatever research is conducted abroad by emigrant physicians has little relevance to the major health problems in their homelands.

4. Foreign-exchange earnings from the remittances of emigrants may play an important role in the balance of payments of some developing countries. However, existing statistics do not indicate what proportion of such remittances is attributable to less-skilled emigrants and what proportion to highly skilled emigrants, either as a whole or grouped according to profession. Professional groups are more likely than less-skilled laborers to take their families with them when they emigrate, so that their remittances might be negligible.

5. The stockpiling of talent abroad until its use can be economically afforded at home could be considered a reasonable, and even desirable, short-term consequence of migration except for the probability that, once absorbed by the host country, the migrants will be reluctant to be repatriated even if offered special incentives. Moreover, when, if ever, the home country is able to afford the return of those abroad, the adaptation of those concerned, both culturally and professionally, may be too far advanced to allow their readaptation to the home country.

These are some of the broad lines of thought expressed in the literature with regard to the consequences of migration. Some researchers measure losses and gains in monetary terms. Others have attempted to measure the impact of migration on health care. In the following sections some of the findings of such studies are presented, along with the difficulties encountered in measuring the consequences of migration. To these findings are added some from the WHO multinational study, as well as analyses developed particularly for this book.

Economic Losses and Gains—A Global View

Those who complain about the consequences of health-manpower migration may couch their arguments in economic terms, often with little understanding of what is implied by the facts and figures they bring to bear on the argument. Similarly, proposals for compensatory payments by the countries of immigration to the countries of emigration generally presuppose the existence of an accurate technique for balancing the account. But this is far from being the case.

There are two major considerations involved in calculating losses and gains (monetary or other) through the migration of health manpower, namely: (1) Which factors are to be taken into account in determining the value of the physician or nurse who migrated? (2) Who are the beneficiaries and who are the deprived, and what did they gain or lose, financially or otherwise?

The difficulties of answering these questions can be illustrated by the following hypothetical case: A young person of Indian ancestry but born in Malaysia, where he received primary and secondary education at the public's expense, decides to study medicine. He goes to Madras, India, for undergraduate medical education and training. His family covers the cost of his tuition and personal expenses during that time. As part of his clinical training, he provides a certain amount of health care to patients in India. Once he obtains his medical degree he returns to Malaysia to practice medicine and, after a few years of rendering services in Malaysia with the medical skills he obtained in India, he moves to Canada for training in a medical specialty. At this point he carries with him the primary and secondary education obtained in Malaysia, the undergraduate medical education obtained in India, and the additional medical experience gained in Malaysia. During the course of his specialty training in Canada, which is paid for by the government of Malaysia, he provides services to patients in Canada. Eventually he migrates to the United States with the total of the knowledge and skills obtained, at a cost in terms of both money and time, in three other countries.

In calculating the value of the physician described above, and thus the losses and gains ensuing from his migration, which factors are to be taken into account? If the physician remains in the United States, to which country or countries could the United States be considered as being indebted? There is also the possibility that, after a few years, with additional training and experience in the United States, the physician will return to Malaysia. If he does so, can Malaysia be considered as owing a debt to India, Canada, and the United States, each of which contributed to the education of the physician while also deriving varying degrees of benefit from the services he provided?

Given the various stages of this physician's career, the following questions arise: Which point in time should be taken into account in determining his value? From which country's perspective should the assessment be made, given that four countries are involved both as contributors to, and recipients of, his skills and knowledge? What would be an appropriate conversion rate to be used in calculating the quantifiable value of the physician? How do unquantifiable factors enter the picture? Second, in each of the countries involved, which specific units (individuals, groups, institutions, and so on) gain or lose as a result of the physician's movement, and what do they gain or lose? Among these, one would need to consider: the migrant himself; the institutions involved in his education; his employers, past and present whether individuals or institutions, private or public; other physicians, whose productivity and therefore value in monetary terms may have either increased or decreased as a result of their access to, or deprivation of, the migrant's assistance; other health workers, whose productivity depends or depended on the supervision given by the migrant; and the country as a whole, that is, the taxpayers, including those who contributed to the migrant's education, those who actually or potentially could have benefited from his services, and those who actually or potentially were deprived of his services.

These are only a few of the factors involved. There are many more, not the least of which would be the problem of relating human-capital flows to other capital flows, including foreign aid and the remittances of the migrants. Also, in instances where the migrants concerned could not be absorbed by the country that produced them, can such migrants be considered a loss to that country? Some would argue that the country, in fact, gains through a partial relief of the unemployment problem, in the sense that such migrants no longer have to be supported at society's expense.

A more pertinent argument is that the migrants themselves constitute no loss, but that the resources invested in them, including time, are lost, in the sense that these resources might have been used in a more profitable way, for example, in the production of larger numbers of health manpower that are cheaper to train and maintain and that would be less inclined to migrate. This is well illustrated by the following list, which shows, for specified geographic entities, the number of one or another type of health personnel that could be produced for the cost of educating one physician:

Thailand [17]
5 nurses or
19 auxiliary sanitarians

East Africa [17]
3 nurses or
15 auxiliary sanitarians or
20 medical assistants or
30 auxiliary nurses

Colombia [17]
8 nurses or
25 auxiliary nurses

Pakistan [16]
4 nurses or
24 medical assistants or
24 lady health visitors or
60 midwives or
60 sanitary inspectors

The simplest method of estimating losses and gains in monetary terms is to determine the cost of producing or replacing those who have migrated. Something approaching this type of calculation has been done with respect to the United States—in one instance by using U.S. $20,000 as the average cost of undergraduate medical education in a developing country and U.S. $83,000 as the average cost in the United States. [61] If these same values are applied to the number of foreign-trained physicians in the United States in 1974 (over 76,000), that country could be considered as having saved over 6 billion dollars by importing physicians trained abroad, and the donor countries as a whole could be considered as having lost over 1.5 billion dollars' worth of medical education—this on the assumption that the physicians remain in the United States.

It is obvious that this type of calculation has severe limitations, in that only one of the many factors previously mentioned is taken into account. Moreover, when viewed from the perspective of individual donor countries, the estimate of U.S. $20,000 as the average cost of undergraduate medical education in the developing countries may be much too high. In Colombia and Sri Lanka, for example, the cost would be closer to one-quarter of that amount, and in Lebanon closer to half. [27, 44] Even from the perspective of the United States, the figure of U.S. $83,000 as the average cost may be too high. A recent study published by the Institute of Medicine indicates U.S. $12,650 per year per student as the average cost in the United States. [62] This would bring the average cost for the four-year period closer to U.S. $50,000 and would reduce the previously cited amount of savings to the United States by nearly half. For such recipient countries as the United Kingdom and the Federal Republic of Germany, the problem of calculating their debt to donor countries in terms of educational costs is compounded by the fact that the migrant physicians include a considerable number who received their medical education in the recipient country—which brings the question back to whether the donor country is the country of birth or the country of graduation.

A study carried out by the United Nations Conference on Trade and Development approaches the problem of assessing losses and gains by focusing on the total net income and the imputed capital value of the migrants, rather than on the cost of their education. [52] That study is based on the assumption that, from the moment of migration, the migrants take with them their productivity and their earning capacity. The recipient countries dealt with in the study are Canada, the United Kingdom, and the United States. Among the populations concerned are physicians, surgeons, and dentists (a total of 46,408) who immigrated to these countries from developing countries during the period 1961–1972. According to the findings of the study, the physicians, surgeons, and dentists involved represent a gross imputed capital value of U.S. $20,551 million and a net income gain of U.S. $18,750 million for the three recipient countries combined.

Other Indicators of Impact—A Global View

Another way of looking at losses and gains is to relate migration both to need, as represented by physician/population ratios, and to the number of years it would take each donor country to replace its emigrant physicians, and each recipient country to produce the equivalent of its foreign physicians.

With respect to the primarily donor countries, the WHO multinational study attempted to measure impact through the development of a composite index reflecting these factors. On the assumption that the index reflects at least a broad order of magnitude of impact, it was found, for example, that Haiti, which lost 534 physicians, suffered twenty-seven times more from that migration than did India, which lost 15,000 (or thirty times more physicians than were lost by Haiti). This is explained by the fact that Haiti would require over ten years to replace its emigrant physicians, as compared with two years for India. Also, among all countries it lost the highest proportion of physicians relative to stock.

While the index, even with its drawbacks, was found to be a useful composite measure of impact, a better understanding of the impact of migration on individual countries was obtained by relating physician emigration, or "loss," to physician coverage, or "need." Through this exercise it was found, for example, that Indonesia and the Republic of Korea, for both of which the impact as measured by the composite index was practically the same, had different problems. Whereas Indonesia had lost only 5 percent of its physicians, it was left with only 0.4 physicians per 10,000 population, and thus its need for physicians was very great. The Republic of

Korea, on the other hand, had lost 19 percent of its physicians but was still left with 4.5 physicians per 10,000 population. In terms of ability to recover from the loss, the Republic of Korea was again found to be better off in that it would need only half a year to replace its lost physicians, as opposed to the four-and-one-half years needed by Indonesia.

In terms of replacement time, the WHO study found that the gain to the recipient country as a result of physician migration was greater than the loss to the donor. On the average, it would take a donor country one year to replace its migrant nationals, while it would take the average recipient country 6.7 years to replace its foreign physicians (on the assumption that production rates remain the same as during the 1960s). This difference holds for developed and developing countries alike, but is in each case worse for the latter, as is shown in the following table:

	Average replacement time in years		
Countries	*All*	*Developed*	*Developing*
Donors	1.0	0.4	2.3
Recipients	6.7	6.6	8.0

Thus, whereas it would take the developed donor, on the average, only 0.4 years to replace its emigrant physicians and the developed recipient 6.6 years to replace its foreign physicians, it would take the developing donor 2.3 years to replace its emigrant physicians and the developing recipient 8.0 years to replace its foreign physicians.

Impact of Physician Migration to the United States

The WHO multinational study covered all countries, including all recipients as well as all donors of physicians. No attempt was made, however, to isolate the movement to the United States alone in terms of the impact it reflected in donor countries, although an attempt was made to summarize the findings of other studies with regard to the impact of that migration in the United States. The following discussion focuses separately on these two aspects of physician migration to the United States.

Impact in Donor Countries

While the United States is the recipient of about half of the world's migrant physicians, the proportion of each country's migrant physicians found in the United States in the early 1970s varied greatly. Table 4-1 shows, for example: that less than 1 percent of the migrant physicians from Malaysia went to the United States, compared with 100 percent from Honduras; that

17 percent of those from Bulgaria, compared with 87 percent of those from Romania, went to the United States; and that 25 percent of those from Paraguay, compared with 93 percent of those from Peru, followed that path. Thus, while the United States had dipped relatively deeply into the pool of physicians in some countries, in others the depletion of the pool had little to do with the United States. On a worldwide basis, about 5 percent of physician stock migrated, with the United States being responsible for about half the depletion of world stock represented by the 5 percent.

The extent of the impact of migration to the United States on each country's domestic stock varied greatly between different countries and

Table 4-1
Foreign Medical Graduates in the United States in 1972, by Region and Country of Graduation, Compared with Total Physician Emigration from Countries

	Emigrant Physicians			
	Estimated Number			
Region and Country of Graduation	*Abroad (1)*	*United States (2)*[a]	*Number in United States as Percentage of all Emigrants from Country of Graduation (3)*[b]	*Number in United States as Percentage of Stock in Country of Graduation (4)*
Americas				
Argentina	1,734	1,536	89	3
Bolivia	199	188	94	9
Brazil	624	497	80	1
Canada	6,726	6,411	95	18
Chile	340	257	95	6
Colombia	1,246	1,161	93	11
Costa Rica	36	26	72	2
Cuba	3,060	2,999	98	43
Dominican Republic	752	722	96	32
Ecuador	193	183	95	8
El Salvador	181	128	71	13
Guatemala	152	135	89	11
Haiti	534	391	73	95
Honduras	65	65	100	9
Mexico	1,718	1,622	94	4
Nicaragua	116	96	83	8
Panama	49	29	59	3
Paraguay	422	105	25	9
Peru	808	754	93	9
Uruguay	96	66	69	2
Venezuela	275	222	81	2
West Indies	263	83	32	7

[a] Figures are estimates of numbers excluding U.S.-born FMGs.

[b] Column 3 = column 2 ÷ column 1.

Table 4-1 continued

Region and Country of Graduation	Emigrant Physicians: Estimated Number Abroad (1)	Estimated Number United States (2)	Number in United States as Percentage of all Emigrants from Country of Graduation (3)	Number in United States as Percentage of Stock in Country of Graduation (4)
Asia				
Afghanistan	25	24	96	2
China (excluding Taiwan)	1,442	644	45	?
China's Prov. of Taiwan	1,884	1,544	82	35
Hong Kong	551	132	24	6
India	15,007	6,303	42	5
Indonesia	250	149	60	3
Iran	3,709	2,082	56	22
Iraq	583	283	41	5
Israel	454	281	62	4
Japan	1,112	1,028	92	1
Lebanon	916	716	78	32
Malaysia	570	5	1	0
Pakistan and Bangladesh	3,319	1,152	35	6
Philippines	9,452	8,846	94	63
Republic of Korea	2,932	2,729	93	18
Republic of South Vietnam	105	25	24	1
Singapore	202	40	20	3
Sri Lanka	872	263	30	8
Syrian Arab Republic	811	270	33	16
Thailand	1,458	1,336	92	27
Turkey	1,943	985	51	6
Europe				
Austria	2,027	1,486	73	11
Belgium	683	384	56	2
Bulgaria	389	65	17	0
Czechoslovakia	1,792	716	40	2
Denmark	161	92	57	1
Finland	96	42	44	1
France	1,399	592	42	1
German Democratic Republic	744	651	87	2
Germany, Federal Republic of	4,560	3,129	69	3
Greece	1,702	873	51	6
Hungary	1,352	868	64	4

Table 4-1 continued

Region and Country of Graduation	Emigrant Physicians: Estimated Number Abroad (1)	Estimated Number United States (2)	Number in United States as Percentage of all Emigrants from Country of Graduation (3)	Number in United States as Percentage of Stock in Country of Graduation (4)
Iceland	76	49	64	16
Ireland	4,308	860	20	24
Italy	2,440	1,973	81	2
Netherlands	624	519	83	3
Norway	112	56	50	1
Poland	1,761	747	42	1
Portugal	264	116	44	1
Romania	455	395	87	1
Spain	2,076	1,398	67	3
Sweden	137	67	49	1
Switzerland	1,377	1,206	88	12
United Kingdom	8,256	2,073	25	3
Yugoslavia	1,482	493	33	2
Africa				
Egypt	2,461	1,006	41	5
Nigeria	418	62	15	5
South Africa	1,662	412	25	4
Sudan	68	3	4	0
Oceania				
Australia	2,238	384	17	2
New Zealand	766	100	13	3
USSR	1,242	782	63	0

Sources (column 1): World Health Organization, *Multinational Study of the International Migration of Physicians and Nurses: Statistical Enquiry* (unpublished information); (column 2): American Medical Association, Center for Health Services Research and Development, *Foreign Medical Graduates in the United States, 1970,* ed. J.N. Haug and B.C. Martin (Chicago: American Medical Association, 1971); (column 4): stock figures from World Health Organization, *World Health Statistics Annual 1972,* vol. 3 (Geneva: World Health Organization, 1976).

regions (table 4–1 and table 4–2). For example, while the United States' share of Argentina's stock was 3 percent, its share of Colombia's stock was 11 percent. Of the Asian countries, 5 percent of India's stock was lost to the United States, compared with 63 percent for the Philippines. The United States' share of migrant physicians had the least impact on the countries of Europe, Oceania, and the USSR, and the greatest on the countries of Asia followed, in turn, by those of the Americas and Africa. The following is a summary (together with comments) for each region, regarding the percentage of physician stock lost to the United States by each country.

Americas

High loss (over 20 percent):	Haiti, Cuba, Dominican Republic
Medium loss (10–20 percent):	Canada, Colombia, El Salvador, Guatemala
Low loss (5–9 percent):	Bolivia, Chile, Ecuador, Honduras, Nicaragua, Paraguay, Peru, West Indies
Lowest loss (less than 5 percent):	Argentina, Brazil, Costa Rica, Mexico, Panama, Uruguay, Venezuela

Among the low-impact countries, the impact is low for two different reasons. In the cases of Argentina, Brazil, and Venezuela, even though the proportion of their emigrant physicians who went to the United States was high (80 percent or more), the impact was still low because the total migration from those countries was relatively low. On the other hand, in the case of Paraguay and the West Indies, the low impact may be accounted for partly by the fact that the proportion who went to the United States was less than one-third of all emigrant physicians. It is known that quite a few Paraguayan physicians migrated to other Latin American countries, and that physicians from the West Indies largely migrated to the United Kingdom and Canada.

Asia

High loss (over 20 percent):	China's Province of Taiwan, Iran, Lebanon, Philippines, Thailand
Medium loss (10–20 percent):	Republic of Korea, Syrian Arab Republic
Low loss (5–9 percent):	Hong Kong, India, Iraq, Pakistan/ Bangladesh, Sri Lanka, Turkey
Lowest loss (less than 5 percent):	Afghanistan, Indonesia, Israel, Japan, Malaysia, Singapore, Republic of South Vietnam

With respect to the low-impact countries, a pattern similar to that for the Americas can be observed with Asian countries. In the case of Japan, for example, the total migration was relatively low, while in the case of India a relatively small proportion of emigrant physicians went to the United States. For half the Asian countries listed, a smaller proportion went to the United States than elsewhere. Physicians from the Commonwealth

Table 4-2
Foreign Medical Graduates in the United States in 1972, by Region of Graduation, Compared with Total Physician Emigration from Countries of the Region

	Emigrant Physicians			
	Estimated Number		*Number in United States as Percentage of All Emigrants from Region of Graduation*	*Number in United States as Percentage of Stock in Region of Graduation*
Region of Graduation	*Abroad (1)*[a]	*In United States (2)*[b]	*(3)*	*(4)*
Africa	5,761	1,486	26	3
Americas	19,767	11,265	57	6
Asia	48,208	28,792	60	8
Europe	40,075	18,856	47	3
Oceania	3,077	484	16	2
USSR	1,242	782	63	0
Origin unknown	14,260	0	0	0
World	132,300	61,665	47	3

Source: Table 4-1.
[a]Includes physicians outside their own country but within their own region.
[b]Excludes U.S.-born FMGs. World figures exclude the mainland of China.

countries of Asia (such as India, Pakistan, Malaysia, Hong Kong, Singapore, and Sri Lanka) prefer to migrate to other Commonwealth countries, chiefly to the United Kingdom but also to Canada, Australia, and New Zealand.

Europe

High loss (over 20 percent):	Ireland
Medium loss (10–20 percent):	Austria, Iceland, Switzerland
Low loss (5–9 percent):	Greece
Lowest loss (less than 5 percent):	All other countries

The high impact on Ireland is not surprising, given that Ireland's total loss of medical graduates was 121 percent of stock. Many of Ireland's graduates are not, however, Irish nationals. Switzerland's medium loss also reflects a sizable portion of graduates who are not Swiss. For Europe as a whole, less than half its emigrant physicians were in the United States. Most of the remainder had gone from one European country to another, or to Canada.

> *Africa and Oceania.* Most migrant physicians from Africa and Oceania went to countries other than the United States, and thus the United States is accountable for only a small proportion of the loss of physicians by those regions. Physicians from Australia and New Zealand tended to migrate between the two countries or, alternatively, to go to other Commonwealth countries, as did many Asians and Africans.

It has been hypothesized that, in donor countries, the loss of physicians through migration results in an even more unequal distribution of physicians between urban and rural areas than is generally the case. With factors such as geographic maldistribution, however, it is difficult to separate cause from effect, since such factors are basically symptomatic of low income and development levels and thus may constitute both cause and effect or perhaps neither. It could be argued that physician coverage of the urban poor and rural populations is low because physicians emigrate, but it could just as well be argued that physicians emigrate because conditions in rural areas and certain urban areas are so poor that no acceptable employment opportunities exist there. The process is part of the vicious circle of poverty, underdevelopment, and disease in which many of the donor countries are trapped.

One line of thought is that, as more and more physicians crowd into urban areas, some of them will be forced, through the resultant shortage of employment opportunities, to seek employment in urderserved areas. In a free-market system, this is unlikely to occur to any appreciable extent as long as no attempt is made to change those conditions in the underserved areas that made them unpalatable to physicians in the first place. Moreover, even if emigration were forbidden, physicians might prefer to take up employment outside the health sector rather than move to such areas.

The WHO study found that, in a number of countries, new graduates were compelled to serve for one or more years in an area of hardship. In some cases but not in others incentives were offered, incentives varying from country to country and including such benefits as free housing, transportation facilities, higher pay, and permission to devote part of the physician's professional time to private practice on a fee basis. It would appear that in many cases compulsory service only postponed the date of emigration. Physicians who leave a country because their only opportunity to practice at home lies in a hardship area are not likely to seek, by choice, work in a similar area in another country. Thus, in the recipient country the deprived often continue to be deprived, while in the donor country they are probably no less deprived than before.

Impact in the United States

In the United States, a team of researchers reviewed the literature pertaining to the quality of care delivered by FMGs with a view toward making recommendations for the future use of such graduates in the United States. The review revealed that, in general, the quality of care might be measurable in three different ways:

1. by focusing on structural variables that could be related quantitatively to one another and to the population served (for example, the characteristics of facilities, of health manpower, or of other components of the health-care-delivery system);
2. by focusing on process measures, that is, on what is done to or for a patient with respect to his particular disease or complaint, and on how well it is done;
3. by focusing on outcome measures, that is, on what happened to the patient in terms of palliation, cure, rehabilitation, or whatever other outcomes are applicable, to determine whether the health status of the individual was improved (or stabilized) by the medical care provided. [63]

All three methods are oriented primarily, if not exclusively, toward the assessment of technical medical care. The first method, which is the most indirect of the three and therefore perhaps the least valid for the purpose intended, was said to be the one most frequently used.

The structural variables most frequently used to measure the level of care provided by physicians were: age, type of graduate medical education, licensure status, specialty, and specialty-board-certification status. With regard to FMGs, additional variables were: native language and culture, language of undergraduate medical education, and status of certification by the ECFMG. According to the authors of the review, the conclusions about FMGs that might be derived from data on these structural variables are mixed, partly because the relationships between structural variables and quality of care are ambiguous. At the same time, the authors felt it would not be unreasonable to conclude that the cumulative weight of the evidence supports the contention that *some* FMGs, particularly the less-than-fully-licensed group and the group at the beginning of their graduate medical training, are more likely to provide lower-quality care than their counterparts who were educated in the United States. This conclusion is based primarily on one or more of three persistent themes: apparent deficiencies in clinical training, beginning at the level of undergraduate medical education abroad and continuing through at least some graduate training programs in the United States; difficulties with the English language; and apparent deficits in the achievements of professional credentials according to U.S. standards. The authors also warn that this contention should not be extended to all FMGs—that the failure to distinguish among different types of FMGs has for too long led to the belief that all FMGs are alike and that those FMGs who have become successful, fully qualified providers are still more similar to the less-than-fully-qualified FMGs on the periphery of the medical profession than to their fully qualified colleagues who trained in the United States.

The authors of the review state that a few studies were carried out with the second method, the use of process measures. For the most part, however, these studies were said to be hampered by the fact that the samples used were too small to contain an adequate representation of the diverse elements of the FMG population. No data were available on the third method, which is much more complex than the other two and involves many factors, some of them independent of the behavior of the physician.

A somewhat different view point emerges from another study in the United States, which focused on an evaluation of policy-related research. Part of the study was devoted to a review, first, of the concepts underlying the various measures used to assess the competence of FMGs and, second, of the published evidence on the technical adequacies and validities of these measures. [34] While that study found that many of the more commonly cited indicators of FMG competence are biased and unreliable, the research evidence indicates that, when properly analyzed, peer-rating studies, as well as data on the performance of FMGs in the ECFMG examination and the FLEX licensure examination, are conceptually and empirically defensible indicators of FMG competence. Taken together, the peer-rating and ECFMG-test data indicate convincingly that, by U.S. standards, FMGs are far less knowledgeable than USMGs about contemporary clinical sciences and techniques, and that the ECFMG-test data do predict clinical proficiency during the early years of practice. There is no evidence as to whether or not these test scores also predict patient welfare. Of the FMGs who passed the screening examinations (ECFMG, FLEX, Board), half or more did so by very few points. There is no evidence or conceptual reason to distinguish the many FMGs who score close to but above 75 (and thus qualify for full licensure) from those who score just under 75 and are not licensed, but are nevertheless providing physician services in the United States. According to the team who conducted this study, the real problem, perhaps a serious one, centers on all FMGs whose pass rate is near the minimum. The team was careful to point out, however, that it has not been definitely shown that such FMGs deliver inferior care or compromise patient welfare. Nor did the team feel there was any evidence or compelling reason to argue that a reduced reliance on FMGs would advance the public interest; the question is whether a marginally competent FMG is better for the patient than no physician at all.

This study examined and evaluated the various methodologies used to assess the impact of FMGs on the quality of care given in the United States.

Among the many studies examined was one on licensure, competence, and manpower distribution. [24] This eight-year follow-up study of a group of USMGs and FMGs challenges the notion that, because a greater proportion of USMGs than of FMGs are licensed, the former show greater medical competence. The research team found that factors unrelated to competence (namely, visa/citizenship status and the state where the licensing examination is administered) are associated with the holding of a license. According to the authors of that report, the closer the FMG is to citizenship status in the United States, the greater the probability of his being licensed. They also state that some of the differences in licensure rates might be explained by differential bureaucratic treatment of FMGs, as compared to USMGs, in the licensing process. State licensing boards are not only arbiters of competence but also de facto manpower-planning agencies. The introduction of the limited license, now in use in forty-three states, points up the manpower-planning function of licensure. Holders of the limited license are restricted to working in areas designated by the licensing board—usually areas experiencing a severe shortage of physicians. According to the authors of the report, the strategy of attracting large numbers of FMGs, licensing relatively few of them, and allowing the unlicensed among them to work only in certain institutions (usually state, municipal, or county hospitals) could allow certain states to ease the critical shortage of physicians in such institutions. One result of this strategy would be a high proportion of unlicensed FMGs, since they are available, are reasonably flexible in terms of the specialties and types of post they will accept, and are often in a vulnerable position because of visa status. As an addendum to the subject of the validity of licensure rates as a measure of the competence of FMGs, the authors of the report suggest that, while the ready availability of such a reservoir of health manpower gives individual states flexibility in their responses to perceived shortages, it also weakens the will to carry out effective long-term medial-manpower planning in the United States.

Another concern in the United States has centered on the question of whether, and to what extent, foreign physicians either worsen or ameliorate the distribution of physicians geographically, institutionally, and by modes of practice and specialties.

With respect to geographic location, available data indicate that FMGs have tended to gravitate to areas where the physician-to-population ratio was already high. Of the more than 74,000 FMGs in the United States in 1972 (including those trained in Canada), about 52,000 or 70 percent were located in the northeastern states—those along the Atlantic seaboard from Maine to the District of Columbia, and those bordering the Great Lakes. By far the heaviest concentration was in New York, the location for 26 percent of all FMGs in 1972. States in which FMGs represented at least one-third of the total stock of physicians in the respective state were: New York, Rhode Island, Delaware, New Jersey, and Illinois. Those in which they represented between one-quarter and one-third of the stock were West Virginia, Michigan, Ohio, Connecticut, and Maryland. [5] The states with the lowest proportions of FMGs tended to be those in the midwest.

Table 4-3 shows that, on the average, the United States had 15.4 active physicians per 10,000 population in 1974. There was, however, a difference of 16.5 physicians per 10,000 population between the best-served state

Table 4-3
Distribution of Foreign Medical Graduates in the United States, by States Ranked according to Proportion of State's Physicians Who Are Foreign Graduates, 1973

State	Proportion of FMGs in State's Physician Pool (%) (1)	Physicians per 10,000 Population: Including FMGs (2)	Physicians per 10,000 Population: Excluding FMGs (3)	Index[a] of Urban Concentration of FMGs (4)
New York	39	24.5	14.9	1.58
New Jersey	35	16.3	10.7	1.57
Rhode Island	34	18.2	12.0	1.32
Delaware	33	14.7	9.8	0.77
Illinois	33	16.0	10.7	1.54
West Virginia	30	11.8	8.3	0.76
Ohio	27	14.2	10.3	1.44
Michigan	26	13.6	10.0	1.99
Maryland	26	25.4	19.0	1.31
Connecticut	23	21.0	16.2	2.71
Florida	20	15.8	12.6	1.38
Missouri	20	9.7	7.8	1.85
Hawaii	19	16.4	13.3	1.12
Pennsylvania	18	16.1	13.2	1.21
Maine	17	12.5	10.4	0.88
Massachusetts	17	22.8	19.0	3.52
Virginia	15	15.2	12.9	1.39
Wisconsin	15	13.2	11.2	0.98
North Dakota	15	10.5	9.0	0.41
New Hampshire	15	14.9	12.7	1.82
Iowa	13	10.8	9.4	1.01
South Dakota	13	8.9	7.8	0.27
Kentucky	12	11.8	10.4	1.64

[a]Index represents percentage of FMGs in stock in urban areas divided by percentage of FMGs in stock in rural areas. If the index is higher than 1, FMG concentration is in urban areas; if lower, in rural areas.

Table 4-3 continued

State	Proportion of FMGs in State's Physician Pool (%) (1)	Physicians per 10,000 Population: Including FMGs (2)	Physicians per 10,000 Population: Excluding FMGs (3)	Index[a] of Urban Concentration of FMGs (4)
Kansas	12	13.4	11.8	1.40
Texas	12	13.7	12.1	1.80
Indiana	12	10.8	9.5	1.01
Minnesota	11	16.7	14.9	1.72
Georgia	10	13.0	11.6	0.87
Arizona	10	17.0	15.3	1.30
Tennessee	9	13.5	12.3	3.19
New Mexico	8	13.4	12.3	1.02
Washington	8	16.9	15.6	1.20
California	8	21.2	18.0	2.30
Vermont	7	18.8	17.4	0.64
Louisiana	6	13.1	12.3	2.12
North Carolina	6	12.5	11.7	1.25
Oklahoma	6	11.0	10.3	1.08
Alabama	6	10.0	9.5	3.88
South Carolina	6	11.2	10.6	2.72
Colorado	5	19.0	18.0	2.24
Nebraska	5	12.8	12.1	3.94
Wyoming	5	10.9	10.4	?
Montana	5	11.5	11.0	0.42
Alaska	5	12.6	12.0	0.59
Oregon	5	16.1	15.4	2.62
Mississippi	4	9.7	9.3	2.48
Nevada	4	12.1	11.6	1.60
Utah	3	15.6	15.1	5.33
Arkansas	2	10.0	9.8	2.00
Idaho	2	9.8	9.6	1.00

Sources (columns 1 and 4): American Medical Association, Center for Health Services Research and Development, *Socioeconomic Issues of Health, 75-76,* ed. H.R. Mason (Chicago: American Medical Association, 1976); (column 2): United States Department of Health, Education, and Welfare, Public Health Service, Health Resources Administration, National Center for Health Statistics, *Health Resources Statistics Reported from the National Center for Health Statistics 1975* (Rockville, Md.: U.S. Department of Health, Education, and Welfare, 1976), and United States Department of Commerce, Bureau of the Census, *Statistical Abstract of the United States, 1975: National Data Book and Guide to Sources* (Washington, D.C.: U.S. Department of Commerce, 1976); (column 3): from columns 1 and 2.

Notes: Columns 1 and 4 refer to 31 December 1973; column 2 refers to 1974. Totals cover active physicians, and graduates of Canadian schools are counted with USMGs.

(Maryland, with 25.4) and the least-served state (South Dakota, with 8.9). If FMGs are excluded from these figures, the physician coverage for Maryland drops from 25.4 to 19.0, a difference of 6.4, while that for South Dakota drops to 7.8, a difference of 1.1. Thus, the difference between the best- and the least-served states is reduced from 16.5 to 11.2. On this basis it is possible to hypothesize that one-third of the inequality between states is caused by FMGs. Figure 4-1, which is based on table 4-3, shows how the spread of states classified by physician coverage is widened when FMGs are added to indigenous stock.

The tendency of FMGs to go to states that already have a high physician/population ratio is not considered to be related to physician income, given that, if anything, there is a tendency for average physician income to vary inversely with the physician/population ratio in the nation's major regions. The following table shows the number of physicians per 10,000 population and the median income of physicians by region and major metropolitan area in 1970. [19]

Region and Area	*Physicians per 10,000 Population, 1970*	*Median Income of Physicians, 1970 (dollars)*
Northeast	18.8	40,000
New York City	27.9	38,700
North Central	12.9	46,100
Chicago	17.0	41,600
South	12.1	45,500
Atlanta	16.2	41,000
West	16.6	42,600
Los Angeles	20.2	47,100
United States	14.8	42,800

Thus, while the northeast and west ranked highest in physician/population ratios in 1970, they ranked lowest in average physician income. While physician income in itself may not be a determinant of physician location, there is considerable evidence that the distribution of federal subsidies with respect to Medicaid, Medicare, and research favors the best-served states and thus encourages the movement of physicians, including FMGs, to such states. This aspect of distribution was discussed more fully in chapter 3.

A longitudinal study of FMGs shows that, although they initially inclined toward areas with low need, their interstate movements tended to be toward areas of greater need. [14] However, because additional FMGs arrived each year and only 8 percent of the cohort studied had moved within a two-year period, the maldistribution between states had failed to improve.

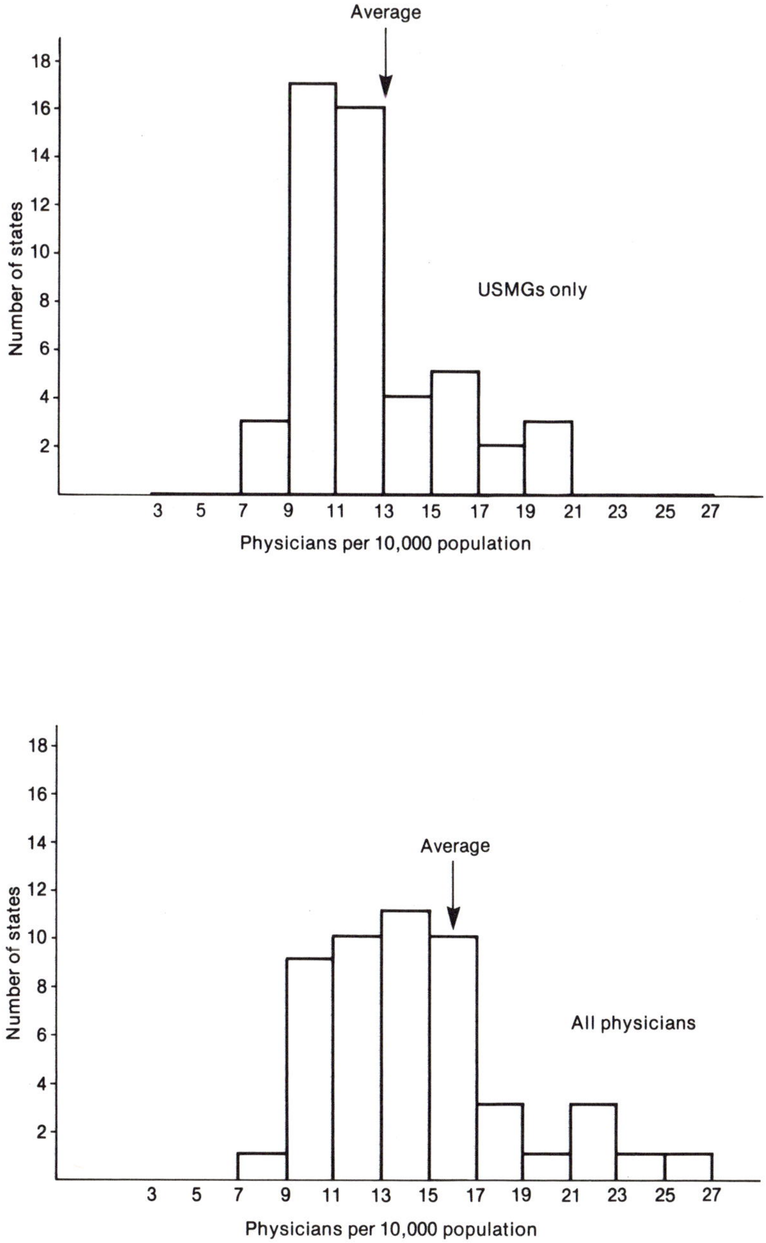

Source: Table 4-3.

Figure 4-1. Distribution of Fifty States of the United States, by Size of Physician Coverage.

Within states, FMGs aggravate urban-rural differentials by their tendency to settle in large metropolitan areas. Table 4-4 shows that, in 1973, whereas 25 percent of the population of the United States resided in nonmetropolitan areas, only 14 percent of USMGs and 8 percent of FMGs were located in such areas. As shown in the following table, the degree of urban concentration was almost twice as high for FMGs as for USMGs.

	Physicians per 10,000 Population (1973)		
	USMGs	*FMGs*	*All*
Metropolitan areas	14.2	3.6	17.8
Nonmetropolitan areas	6.9	0.8	7.7
Total	12.4	3.0	15.4
Ratio of metropolitan to nonmetropolitan	2.1	4.5	2.3

By comparison, ten years earlier, in 1963, the number of active nonfederal physicians per 10,000 population was 4.6 in the more isolated rural areas, as compared with 17.3 (or nearly four times as many) in the larger metropolitan areas. The national average was 12.5, with the number in metropolitan and adjacent areas as a whole being 13.6, and that in nonmetropolitan areas being 7.5. [22] Thus, whereas the national average rose by 2.9 physicians per 10,000 population, the number in metropolitan areas as a whole rose by 4.2 and that in nonmetropolitan areas by 0.2. The changes from 1963 to 1973 are summarized in the following table.

	Physicians per 10,000 Population		
Year	*Average*	*Metropolitan*	*Nonmetropolitan*
1963	12.5	13.6	7.5
1973	15.4	17.8	7.7
Difference over 10 years	+2.9	+4.2	+0.2

The thousands of FMGs who joined the pool of physicians in the United States during the ten-year period thus aggravated the very precarious imbalance existing in 1963.

A study of FMGs in the United States in 1970 indicated that those from India and Thailand showed the greatest propensity to practice in metropolitan areas (97 percent in each case). On the other hand, countries having a relatively high proportion of their graduates located in nonmetropolitan areas included Spain (45 percent), Dominican Republic (27 percent),

Table 4–4
Distribution of Active Physicians in the United States, by Area of Location, 1973

	Total (100%)	Metropolitan Areas		Nonmetropolitan Areas	
		Number	*Percentage*	*Number*	*Percentage*
1. Active physicians	319,567	278,672	87	40,895	13
2. FMGs	60,817	56,359	92	4,458	8
3. USMGs	258,750	222,313	86	36,437	14
4. U.S. resident population (thousands) in December 1972	209,448	156,922	75	52,526	25
5. USMGs per 10,000 population	12.4	14.2		6.9	
6. All physicians	15.2	17.8		7.7	

Sources (row 1): American Medical Association, Center for Health Services Research and Development, *Socioeconomic Issues of Health, 75–76,* ed. H.R. Mason (Chicago, American Medical Association, 1976); (row 2): based on data in American Medical Association, *Socioeconomic Issues*; (row 3): residuals; (row 4): United States Department of Health, Education, and Welfare, Public Health Service, Health Resourses Administration, Bureau of Health Planning and Resources Development, *Trends Affecting U.S. Health Care System*, DHEW Publication no. (HRA) 76.14503 (Rockville, Md.: U.S. Department of Health, Education, and Welfare, 1976).

Note: Row 2 excludes graduates of Canadian schools.

Mexico (19 percent), and Cuba (17 percent)—all Spanish-speaking countries. [3]

Table 4–5 shows the distribution of FMGs, as a percentage of all active physicians in the United States in 1973, by size of geographic location and by mode of practice. The proportion of stock represented by FMGs was nearly twice as high in metropolitan areas as in rural areas (20 percent and 11 percent, respectively). In very large urban areas, FMGs constituted one-third of all physicians and half of all hospital staff. The urban-rural differential in the proportion of FMGs was greatest for office-based physicians and for interns and residents. With regard to the largest urban areas, this differential was 3.0 for all modes of practice, 2.7 for office-based practice, 3.0 for interns and residents, and 2.0 for hospital staff. This differential probably arises because hospitals are usually located in densely populated (urban) areas, and there are thus relatively few hospital-based openings in the less densely populated, nonurban areas.

Although FMGs appear to have worsened the geographic distribution of physicians in the United States, they also appear to have become the saviors of the nonaffiliated hospital, at least insofar as house-staff positions are concerned. This is shown in table 4–6, which presents data on FMGs holding house-staff positions, by medical-school affiliation, in 1960 and

1970. The difference in the proportion of positions held by FMGs during the two years is summarized below.

	Percentage of House-Staff Positions Held by FMGs in:		
Year	*All Hospitals*	*Affiliated Hospitals*	*Nonaffiliated Hospitals*
1960	26	17	38
1970	32	27	61
Difference	+6	+10	+23

Thus, whereas the total number of house-staff positions held by FMGs was only 6 percent greater in 1970 than in 1960, the number was 23 percent greater in nonaffiliated hospitals, compared to 10 percent greater in affiliated hospitals. Not only were more FMGs being concentrated in nonaffiliated hospitals, but this concentration occurred in a diminishing number of nonaffiliated hospitals. While the number of positions filled in all hospitals grew by 39 percent in the period 1960–1970, the rate of growth was not uniform between affiliated and nonaffiliated hospitals: The number of posi-

Table 4–5
Urban/Rural Distribution of Foreign Medical Graduates in the United States, by Modes of Practice, 1973

	FMGs as a Percentage of all Physicians			
Number of Inhabitants in Area	*Total*	*Office-Based*	*Interns and Residents*	*Full-Time Hospital Staff*
Total in United States	19	13	33	31
All rural areas	11	9	17	24
< 10,000	9	8	0	26
10,000–24,999	9	7	13	25
25,000–49,999	11	9	44	29
All metropolitan areas	20	14	33	32
50,000–499,999	11	8	17	22
500,000–999,999	19	13	31	31
1,000,000–4,999,999	19	13	30	28
5,000,000 +	33	24	50	50

Source: American Medical Association, Center for Health Services Research and Development, *Socioeconomic Issues of Health, 75–76*, ed. H.R. Mason (Chicago: American Medical Association, 1976).

Table 4–6
Foreign Medical Graduates Serving as House Staff in U.S. Hospitals, by Medical-School Affiliation and Size of Hospital, 1960 and 1970

	1960			*1970*		
Affiliation and Size of Hospital	*Total Filled Positions*	*Filled by FMGs*	*Percentage Filled by FMGs*	*Total Filled Positions*	*Filled by FMGs*	*Percentage Filled by FMGs*
Affiliated hospitals						
Total	20,609	3,402	17	43,048	11,587	27
Less than 200 beds	764	179	23	2,374	420	18
200–299	1,864	442	24	1,375	530	39
300–499	4,425	829	19	6,815	2,589	38
500 and over	13,556	1,952	14	17,815	4,923	28
Nonaffiliated hospitals						
Total	15,829	6,055	38	7,724	4,695	61
Less than 200 beds	1,662	914	55	512	265	52
200–299	3,314	1,869	56	1,167	789	68
300–499	5,503	2,059	37	2,208	1,547	70
500 and over	5,350	1,213	23	2,899	1,465	51

Source: R. Stevens and J. Vermeulen, *Foreign Trained Physicians and American Medicine,* DHEW Publication no. (NIH) 73-325 (Bethesda, Md.: U.S. Department of Health, Education, and Welfare, 1972).

Notes: Data for 1960 include graduates of Canadian medical schools and exclude American graduates of foreign schools. Data for 1970 refer only to interns and residents in house-staff positions.

tions filled in affiliated hospitals grew by 109 percent, while the number filled in nonaffiliated hospitals decreased by 51 percent. The positions filled in affiliated hospitals accounted for 85 percent of all filled positions in 1970, as opposed to 57 percent in 1960. Thus, as the number of positions in affiliated hospitals increased, they were increasingly taken up by USMGs, while the dwindling number of positions in nonaffiliated hospitals were largely left to FMGs.

With regard to hospital size, it would appear that FMGs find the most accommodation in medium-sized hospitals, both affiliated and nonaffiliated.

As regards specialties, the gaps filled by FMGs are shown in table 4–7. Of the 57,172 residency positions offered in 1974, nearly two-thirds were filled by USMGs. Of the total number of positions offered, only 8 percent remained unfilled, as opposed to the 35 percent that might have remained unfilled had the FMGs not been available.

It has been hypothesized that FMGs largely gravitate to residency positions in such specialties as anesthesiology, pathology, and psychiatry because such positions are less attractive to USMGs. On the assumption that USMGs have priority of choice (which may not be the case) and that, after their choices were made, there were still 20,032 positions left from which the 15,359 FMGs could choose, it is not clear why the FMGs made the choices indicated in table 4–7. Given that FMGs filled an average of 77 percent of the positions left vacant by USMGs (with the result that 4,673 positions were still left unfilled), why did they fill much more than that average in positions such as anesthesiology (84 percent), general practice (84 percent), internal medicine (90 percent), ophthalmology (92 percent), pediatrics (88 percent), surgery (84 percent), and urology (86 percent)? Conversely, why did they not fill more of the available positions in child psychiatry, family practice, radiology (general, diagnostic, and therapeutic), and pathology?

With regard to USMGs, who filled an average of 65 percent of all positions offered, it would appear that, in relation to that average, they were not particularly attracted to positions in anesthesiology (41 percent), child psychiatry (53 percent), general practice (11 percent), pathology (40 percent), physical medicine (24 percent), psychiatry (56 percent), and radiology (except diagnostic radiology, to which they were rather highly attracted). On the other hand, they showed a considerably greater-than-average interest in dermatology (90 percent), family practice (74 percent), neurosurgery (75 percent), ophthalmology (92 percent), orthopedic surgery (86 percent), otolaryngology (79 percent), plastic surgery (76 percent), and urology (76 percent). On the whole, the data on specialties would suggest that FMGs have about the same preferences for certain specialties as do USMGs.

The residency positions offered in 1974 are viewed from another perspective, by type of hospital control, in table 4–8. On the basis of assump-

Table 4–7
Residencies in the United States, by Specialty, 1974

Specialty	Total Positions Offered (Number) (1)	Positions Filled by USMGs (Number) (2)	Positions Filled by USMGs Percentage (3)	Residual Positions (1 – 2) (Number) (4)	Positions Filled by FMGs: Number and as Percentage of Residual — Number (5)	Percentage (6)	Positions Unfilled: Number and as Percentage of Total Offered — Number (7)	Percentage (8)
Anesthesiology	2,260	934	41	1,326	1,110	84	216	10
Child psychiatry	744	393	53	351	177	50	174	23
Colonic and rectal surgery	34	20	59	14	10	71	4	12
Diagnostic radiology	2,300	1,740	76	560	328	59	232	10
Dermatology	778	698	90	80	59	74	21	3
Family practice	3,342	2,457	74	885	212	24	673	20
General practice	333	36	11	297	250	84	47	14
Internal medicine	11,353	8,102	71	3,251	2,922	90	329	3
Neurosurgery	645	484	75	161	123	76	38	6
Neurology	1,124	739	66	385	306	79	79	7
Nuclear medicine	129	60	47	69	34	49	35	27
Obstetrics and gynecology	3,652	2,308	63	1,344	1,113	83	231	6
Ophthalmology	1,579	1,445	92	134	123	92	11	1
Orthopedic surgery	2,454	2,116	86	338	259	77	79	3
Otolaryngology	1,049	826	79	223	168	75	55	5
Pathology	3,404	1,364	40	2,040	1,471	72	569	17
Pathology, forensic	60	18	30	42	10	24	32	53
Neuropathology	66	28	42	38	12	32	26	39
Pediatrics	4,988	3,317	67	1,671	1,467	88	204	4
Pediatric allergology	135	91	67	44	23	52	21	16

Table 4–7 continued

Specialty	Total Positions Offered (Number) (1)	Positions Filled by USMGs (Number) (2)	Positions Filled by USMGs Percentage (3)	Residual Positions (1 – 2) (Number) (4)	Positions Filled by FMGs: Number and as Percentage of Residual — Number (5)	Positions Filled by FMGs — Percentage (6)	Positions Unfilled: Number and as Percentage of Total Offered — Number (7)	Positions Unfilled — Percentage (8)
Pediatric cardiology	142	87	61	55	37	67	18	13
Physical medicine	507	120	24	387	276	71	111	22
Plastic surgery	422	321	76	101	76	75	25	6
Psychiatry	5,012	2,806	56	2,206	1,564	71	642	13
Radiology	900	342	38	558	376	67	182	20
Surgery	7,802	4,996	64	2,806	2,358	84	448	6
Therapeutic radiology	484	220	46	264	154	58	110	23
Thoracic surgery	318	193	61	125	103	82	22	7
Urology	1,156	879	76	277	238	86	39	3
Total	57,172	37,140	65	20,032	15,359	77	4,673	8

Source: American Medical Association, 76th Annual Report, "Medical Education in the United States 1975–1976," appendix 1, *Journal of the American Medical Association* 236(1976):3049–3055.

Note: USMGs include graduates of Canadian schools.

Table 4-8
Residencies in the United States, by Type of Hospital Contract, 1974

	Total Positions Offered	*Positions Filled by USMGs*		*Residual Positions (1 – 2)*	*Positions Filled by FMGs: Number and as Percentage of Residual*		*Positions Unfilled: Number and as Percentage of Total Offered*	
	Number (1)	*Number (2)*	*Percentage (3)*	*Number (4)*	*Number (5)*	*Percentage (6)*	*Number (7)*	*Percentage (8)*
Combined Hospitals	23,008	17,012	74	5,996	4,580	76	1,416	6
Federal								
U.S. Air Force	342	291	85	51	2	4	49	14
U.S. Army	946	870	92	76	23	30	53	6
U.S. Navy	763	683	90	80	11	14	69	9
Public Health Service	165	104	63	61	28	46	33	20
Veterans Administration	1,177	534	45	643	579	90	64	5
Other federal	80	51	64	29	18	62	11	14
Total	3,473	2,533	73	940	661	70	279	8
Governmental nonfederal								
State	5,272	3,235	61	2,037	1,352	66	685	13
County	2,775	1,844	67	931	693	74	238	9
City	1,035	406	39	629	558	89	71	7
City-county	466	318	68	148	88	60	60	13
Hospital district	294	199	68	95	62	65	33	11
Total	9,842	6,002	61	3,840	2,753	72	1,087	11

Table 4–8 continued

	Total Positions Offered	Positions Filled by USMGs		Residual Positions (1 – 2)	Positions Filled by FMGs: Number and as Percentage of Residual		Positions Unfilled: Number and as Percentage of Total Offered	
	Number (1)	Number (2)	Percentage (3)	Number (4)	Number (5)	Percentage (6)	Number (7)	Percentage (8)
Nongovernmental nonprofit								
Church related	3,767	1,782	47	1,985	1,526	77	459	12
Nonprofit corporation	16,731	9,648	58	7,083	5,673	80	1,410	7
Total	20,948	11,430	56	9,068	7,199	79	1,869	9
Proprietary corporation	349	163	47	186	166	89	20	6
Grand total	57,170	37,140	65	20,030	15,359	77	4,671	8

Source: American Medical Association, 76th Annual Report, "Medical Education in the United States 1975-1976," appendix 1, *Journal of the American Medical Association* 236(1976):3049–3055.

Note: Two proprietary-partnership positions offered and not filled by either FMGs or USMGs were omitted from the totals. Thus totals in columns 1 and 8 show 2 less than those in table 4–7.

tions similar to those previously stated, for example, that USMGs have both particular interests and priority of choice, and that FMGs are free to choose among positions left unfilled by USMGs, the question again arises as to why, with 20,030 positions from which to choose and 4,671 positions left unfilled, FMGs made the choices shown in table 4-8.

Given that FMGs filled an average of 77 percent of the positions left vacant by USMGs, why did they fill much more than that average in proprietary-corporation hospitals (89 percent) in governmental nonfederal city hospitals (89 percent), and in Veterans' Administration hospitals (90 percent)? Conversely, why did they fill much less than that average in state, city-county, and hospital-district hospitals, or in public-health services?

With regard to USMGs, who filled an average of 65 percent of all positions offered, it would appear that, in relation to that average, they were not particularly attracted to proprietary-corporation hospitals (47 percent), church-related hospitals (47 percent), nonfederal city hospitals (39 percent), and Veterans' Administration hospitals (45 percent). Conversely, they appeared to be highly attracted to Army, Navy, and Air Force hospitals. Taken altogether, the data suggest that the lower the proportion of positions taken by USMGs in individual hospitals, the higher the proportion of residual vacancies taken by FMGs.

Epilogue Physician Migration in a Global Manpower Market: The United States and the Developing Countries

John H. Bryant
Deputy Assistant Secretary for International Health
Department of Health, Education, and Welfare

The movement of physicians from the less-developed countries (LDCs) to the United States (90,000 in twenty-five years) has probably been the largest migration of medical manpower in history. Migrant physicians represent 5 percent of the world supply of physicians, and half of that migrant pool is now in the United States.

The forces that promote and direct streams of migratory manpower are obviously not peculiar to our time, nor to medicine. Throughout history, man has often traveled in search of more favorable conditions; driven by disappointment, despair, and fear, and drawn by hope, promise, and safety. Each migration has its own characteristics, with one set of factors pushing, another set pulling and often directing. At times, as with war, natural disasters, or starvation, the forces at work are powerful, even brutal, and involve entire populations. At other times the forces are complex, not necessarily insistent in their power, and involve only a segment of a population.

The migration of physicians falls into this second category. The forces are multiple and complex, and the reasons for the decisions of the migrants are often difficult to sort out. The strength and impact of the resultant migration cannot be stated in the same dramatic and explicit terms as in the case of natural disasters, but there is no doubting their power—the number of physicians who have left their own countries and moved to the United States is twice the entire physician population of Africa, and one-half that of Asia. Taking the dual loss—of highly educated manpower (a precious resource in poor countries) and of public monies invested in physician education (between $2 billion and $20 billion, depending on the mode of calculation)—the social cost of the migration could be seen as a major disaster. But is it such a disaster? Since not all resources available for social purposes are put to good use, it would be more realistic to say that, if such resources were well used in the countries of origin, particularly if attention were given to equity in their distribution, the impact on health could be substantial.

In considering the dynamics of the migration, it helps to think in terms of pushing and pulling factors. That may be somewhat simplistic, since the two sides of the equation do not develop independently of one another and then simply interact. Furthermore, the forces acting on this migration are only surface reflections of much larger forces underlying them, including global as well as societal maldistribution of resources, inappropriate technology transfers, institutional weaknesses characteristic of underdevelopment, and so on—a long list.

It is helpful to think of the forces that appear to be at work in the sending nations, and in the United States, and then to reflect on their interaction. But we are interested in more than the dynamics of physician movement. We are concerned about the impact of the migration on the countries of origin and on the United States. We want to know about the public policies that are formed in the donor countries and in the United States in reaction to these large-scale physician migrations. Knowing of recent U.S. legislation designed to limit entry of FMGs, we are curious about the impact of that action at home and abroad. This book has dealt with most of these issues; indeed, the authors' analysis represents a distinct contribution to the field. I will reflect on the points they have made and add some of my own. Finally, I will look briefly at an issue that is largely bypassed in this volume but that may turn out to be important for the United States in the future: the problem of U.S. citizens who go abroad for their medical education and then return home, the U.S. foreign medical graduates (USFMGs).

Migration from the LDCs—Forces and Patterns

In sorting through the various factors that contribute to the migration of physicians, the authors correctly direct attention toward the serious socioeconomic imbalances within and between countries as the most important cause of migration. In the poorest nations, and even in many of those that are not so poor, large segments of the population live in poverty or at a subsistence level, dependent on government resources for social services such as education and health when they are available, but in fact going without them much of the time.

It is easy to overlook the extent of poverty of resources in developing countries and the meaning of this for a professional. The poorer countries have average per-capita incomes of well under U.S. $250, and the meaning of "average" here is that many are pressed deeply below that figure; 800 million people in the developing world live in absolute poverty, with incomes of less than U.S. $50 per year.[1] Resources available for health services are starkly limited: only $1 to $2 per capita per year in most of Africa and Asia.[2] As important as the scarcity is the slowness of change, usually only 2 or 3 percent per year. Those who wait for change within these parameters must wait for generations.[3]

Two extremes of response by the professionals can be envisioned. Some find the situation intolerable: social despair, political instability, inflexible bureaucracies, professional isolation, lack of technological support. They turn away, either by moving as close as possible to social and professional advancement in urban settings at home or by emigrating to a more affluent society abroad. Others also find the situation intolerable, but work to change it, struggling with the problems of underdevelopment, combating the diseases of poverty, trying to extend services to the social periphery. Reality, of course, is more complicated than these two poles of choice. Issues and individual reactions to them cover a vast range of variations and do not permit any simple delineation.

From this range of factors, the authors point out two related to technology transfer that are particularly interesting. One of these has to do with how the elite of the LDCs often contribute to transfers of inappropriate technology and values. The professional, social, and economic elite who, for the most part, hold the reins of power often share the values and tastes of the affluent societies of the more-developed countries (MDCs), and they are often willing partners in transferring and perpetuating these values and the patterns of production and consumption they represent. This idea of "willing partners" calls attention to another problem that frequently appears in negotiation about technology transfer, namely, the interest of both donors and recipients in inappropriate technology—usually in the form of hospital-based, highly sophisticated, superspecialty services and research. Donors and recipients cooperate willingly in the pursuit of these technologies, usually adding to the concentration of investments in urban areas and thereby diverting resources away from primary health services in the periphery. Meanwhile, the poor majority have no advocates at the conference table.

The second factor has to do with the competitive advantages the MDCs have in marketing their products in the developing world. Here, medical education often plays a twisted role. Professional education exported from the MDCs carries the biases of those countries, and usually lacks relevance to the needs of the poorer countries. Professionals educated according to that standard demand the technology that was available to them during the course of their education. Either this demand is met by the developing country, which purchases the technology and thus diverts scarce resources from more appropriate levels of health care, or the professionals migrate to the source of the technology. Thus, the exporters of education and technology either find a ready market abroad or become the recipients of migrant health manpower educated according to their own requirements.

In discussing these and other matters, the authors may be accused of occasionally exaggerating reality. In discussing problems of physician migration, for example, they generalize about health professionals, describing them as elite-oriented, decisions of affluence, and committed to the use of high technology. That caricature often holds, to be sure, but exceptions to it are also important. Many health professionals are committed to the needs of the poor; they fight for the redistribution of resources, work hard for relevance, and urge the development of more appropriate technology.

Similarly, the so-called beneficiaries of inappropriate technology transfer—corporations, academicians, research workers, and medical practitioners—are depicted as absorbing profits, collecting publication credits, living on fellowships, and traveling to many meetings, with little benefit to the poor of the world. Again, the caricature is true much of the time, but it should also be acknowledged that research, publications, fellowships, and meetings are important channels for expanding and sharing knowledge, for promoting self-reliance among the poorer nations, and for developing relevant and effective programs. Indeed, they are often used for these purposes.

Perhaps the most interesting idea developed in the book, one that the authors draw on extensively, is that of *effective economic demand* (EED) for physicians as an explanation of migratory behavior. Effective economic demand is derived from the assumption that a given per-capita gross domestic product will sustain only a given physician density. The authors do not specify the actual quantitative relationship beyond providing figure 3-6 (see p. 109). Estimating from the regression line of this figure, it appears that a per-capita GDP of U.S. $110 to $140 will sustain a physician density of about 1 per 10,000 population, and that this relationship holds for the full range of values depicted.

Countries having a higher level of physician coverage than the theoretical level corresponding to their per-capita GDP tend to lose physicians, and those having a lower level tend to gain physicians. India is an example of the former case and the United States of the latter. India had a level of per-capita GDP in 1970 that could support 0.6 physicians per 10,000 population, but it actually had 2.1 physicians per 10,000. Consistent with the authors' concept, India, in recent years, has been a major source of migrant physicians. The United States, on the other hand, has far fewer physicians than it can economically afford (according to this concept) and also has a large effective economic demand for them.

The authors draw heavily on the concept of the EED. A more analytical treatment of the concept itself would have been interesting. For example, it would be surprising if the relationship between per-capita GDP and density of physicians, as described by the EED, were linear. [Author's note: The relationship is not linear, but is an exponential function in the form: $y = ae^x + b$.] One would expect that the higher incomes of physicians in the MDCs would mean that greater increments of per-capita GDP would be required to sustain the same density of physicians as in the poorer countries.

Such questions notwithstanding, the authors have empirical observations on their side. These relationships between economic development and migratory behavior of physicians hold for almost all countries over a wide range of levels of economic development. Of course, many noneconomic factors are also at work in this area, but the EED appears to be a consistent predictor of migratory behavior.

Using this indicator of market forces, the authors suggest how countries might act in setting public policy concerning manpower production. They point out the folly of increasing physician production to make up for losses through migration when the EED is already too low to sustain the existing number of physicians.

It is common knowledge that, generally, market forces do not serve the poor. Thus, while physician behavior appears to follow market forces, public policy may have to act against those factors. If the pattern of physician behavior is to migrate away from social needs, particularly under conditions of limited economic development, then socially oriented public policy might be used to counter such market effects. The EED concept again reminds us that investment in physician production may be a waste of resources. If physicians who will work in areas of social need are in short supply, then, instead of a simple increase in physician production, alternative approaches to reaching those populations should be pursued. There are a variety of patterns of health manpower that can function effectively with physician shortages. Many countries have been successful in using combinations of auxiliary personnel and community health workers functioning under the leadership of the few health professionals available.

In considering the factors that might be taken into account in developing alternative health-manpower policies, it is useful to know the relative costs of producing physicians and other health personnel. The authors present various data on the costs of medical education, but, as they state, the cost is difficult to estimate and depends on the factors taken into account. My own studies in the mid-1960s revealed an average cost per medical-school graduate of about U.S. $24,000.[4] This figure was arrived at after studying nine schools selected from LDCs on three continents, but it has probably increased considerably since that time. Using such data, countries can calculate the loss in educational investment of annual physician migrations—$2,400,000, for example, in a country losing 100 graduates per year.

Those countries that consider responding to migration by increasing production should recognize that, if 50 percent of their graduates migrate, the cost per graduate remaining in the country is effectively doubled. To go further, the cost in public monies (most of the cost of medical education is paid for with public funds) for placing graduates in locations of social need is usually much higher. For instance, if only one of every ten or twenty graduates work in a location of public need, such as a rural district, the effective cost of placing that graduate there is ten to twenty times the unit cost of production—for example, $250,000 to $500,000. Admittedly, this is a rigorous criterion of cost, since graduates who do not work in locations of need also represent some benefit to the country. The point being emphasized, however, is the cost of achieving the intended social goal.

Those same studies show that in Africa the cost of producing a medical assistant (a medical-care auxiliary with two to three years of training) was about one-twentieth the cost of producing a physician.[5] The cost difference would be even greater when comparing the training and utilizing of community health workers. Generally, those workers receive a few weeks or months of training and work either part-time or as volunteers. Detailed information about comparative costs, specific for the countries concerned, is essential for making sensible choices among alternative health-manpower plans.

A deeper question underlies this discussion of physician migration. What is its importance? Seen as an isolated phenomenon—the human hopes and stresses of the migrants and their families, the frustrations and disappointments of public administrators and educators—the problem has undeniable importance. But in the context of the serious need of developing countries to bring health services to their underserved populations in distant rural and deprived urban settings, which require personnel who are both committed and competent to function in those settings, the migrant problem may be of only marginal importance. As the authors have shown, migrant physicians may not represent a crucial loss to public service; for the most part they are from urban areas of relative excess. So while there is a loss of national resources, the loss is from a population of professionals who are already partly lost to the social needs of the country.

In short, for the LDCs the great challenge is the equitable distribution of health services, using appropriate combinations of paramedical and community health workers together with whatever physicians and other health professionals are available. Promotion of physician education should be seen in relation to the investments of manpower and public monies required, and especially to the wastage due to migration and other career choices that carry physicians away from serving high-priority social needs. Policy-level reactions to physician migration should be tempered with understanding of the limited effectiveness of most of the corrective steps available. Given that many of the forces at work are beyond the control of policy makers, the risk is high that shortsighted solutions, such as increased physician production, with relatively few new graduates serving social priorities, will have only marginal effects.

Migration to the United States and the Impact of Legislation

The forces contributing to the flow of FMGs from the donor countries have analogous forces drawing that migrant stream toward the United States. Some of those forces have been precisely complementary to those in the donor countries, with a high effective economic demand for physicians in the United States matching the low effective economic demand in the donor countries. Others have been peculiar to the United States, emerging from the evolution of its own medical system, such as the emphases on specialization and research. Still others, such as immigration laws and the widespread availability of house-staff positions, have simply facilitated the entry of FMGs. We will examine these forces, and then proceed to consider the public-policy steps being taken in the United States to counteract them.

Four major historical threads came together to form the forces drawing foreign physicians toward the United States. First, the Flexner reform had the effect not only of improving the quality of medical education but also of restricting the numbers of entrants into the physician pool, a limitation long supported by the AMA but ultimately circumvented, at least in part, by the entry of the FMGs.

Second, the rising trend of specialization, away from Flexner's concept of a relatively homogeneous cadre of physicians fitting a safe and competent standard, and toward a variety of specialists with multiple career choices, created multiple avenues of entry for immigrant physicians. The specialization trend was advanced by the strong support provided by the U.S. government for biomedical research in the medical schools. This introduced a research-oriented bias into medical education, with an increased tendency toward specialization. Concomitantly, the research and specialty-oriented medical schools tended to pay relatively little attention to health services, particularly for populations in need, a factor that both added to the perceptions of physician shortages and helped to create opportunities for the expansion of hospitals not affiliated with medical schools.

Third, there was a great expansion in the demand for physicians. This demand had at least two components that were relevant to the entry of foreign physicians: an increasing demand for physicians in general, and a demand that was selective to some extent for the FMGs. The increasing general demand was the product of a number of factors: the rising affluence of the American population; an increasing interest in (some would say dependence on) medical care; and the emergence of new mechanisms for financing medical care, including health insurance on the private side and public financing (especially Medicaid and Medicare) on the government side. These factors coalesced, as the authors point out, to create an effective economic demand well in excess of the available supply of physicians.

Simultaneously, another form of demand was at work creating a special opportunity for FMGs. Following World War II, and continuing over the next two decades, government funds and private philanthropy contributed to a substantial expansion of the hospital system in the United States. That expansion, in turn, created a need for intern and resident physicians that far exceeded the output of the domestic medical schools. This gap between supply and demand was particularly prominent in hospitals unaffiliated with medical schools. Indeed, an oddity in this manpower system is that these nonaffiliated hospitals expanded their training programs for interns and residents largely independently of the availability of domestic-medical-school graduates. In other words, these hospitals needed interns and residents and, without effective access to domestic graduates, that need could be met only by FMGs.

Fourth, given the demand for physicians in the United States, and the push factors at work on foreign physicians abroad, all that was needed to generate and sustain the migratory flow were liberal immigration and licensing regulations. These, too, fell into place. Earlier U.S. programs for encouraging international exchange of students (the Fulbright program, for example) evolved in the Smith-Mundt Act of 1948, which authorized a special category of visa, the Exchange Visa or J visa. This provided a mechanism both for expanding graduate medical education and for meeting the growing need for house staff in hospitals, although neither of these was the intent of the act. Mechanisms for changing from exchange visitor to immigrant status also evolved: In the mid-1960s it was necessary to return home for two years, but beginning in 1970 a direct conversion to immigrant status was possible.

In addition to coming under the Exchange Visitor Program, foreigners could also be admitted directly as immigrants. In 1965 the immigration law was liberalized with respect to professional and highly skilled personnel, thus widening the entryway for foreign physicians. In recent years, the proportion of physicians entering as immigrants has far exceeded the proportion entering as exchange visitors.

While immigration regulations were becoming more liberal, licensing, which is the prerogative of the individual states, became more restrictive. The result was not an absolute barrier to FMGs' practicing, but the development of a variety of modes of licensing: fully licensed; less-fully licensed (a category accepted for practice under certain circumstances, such as in public hospitals); and unlicensed or "underground."

With these several forces at work, a migration of physician manpower without historical precedent was underway, the volume, distribution, and characteristics of which the authors document in analytical detail. Some of those characteristics are particularly interesting in terms of their impact on physician-shortage problems in the United States, and in relation to the congressional action intended to restrict the entry of FMGs.

The FMGs helped to relieve one area of physician shortage—house-staff positions in nonaffiliated hospitals. Many such hospitals had difficulty filling these posts with U.S. graduates, but they could attract FMGs; the latter have made up about 40 percent of residents in city hospitals, church-operated hospitals, and psychiatric hospitals. This distribution was skewed toward nine states, which have 43 percent of all residencies in the United States but 73 percent of FMG-filled residencies. By 1970, overall, 60 percent of residencies in nonaffiliated hospitals were filled by FMGs.[6]

Two sides of the locating of FMGs in those settings can be noted. On the one hand, many of those positions were created to take advantage of the availability of the FMGs, and even to attract them; this calls into question the extent and nature of the shortage. On the other hand, many of those hospitals were in underserved areas and were major sources of care for populations of lower socioeconomic status. It appears, therefore, that FMGs have made substantial contributions during their residencies to health services in underserved areas.

After residency training, however, as the authors show, FMGs have tended to settle in localities where physician-population densities are already high and in specialties that are not in short supply, thus accentuating existing maldistribution. For example, about one-third of the urban-rural imbalance can be attributed to FMGs.

In brief, the FMGs have added substantially to the physician pool in the United States now making up approximately 21 percent of that pool, but their choices of locations and specialties have differed somewhat from those of domestic graduates, tending even more strongly away from shortage areas. Lacking a planned system for health-manpower development, the United States depends largely on market forces to determine the production and distribution of health personnel. The FMGs have responded to those market forces differently than domestic graduates, but there would appear to be no basis for criticizing their choices any more than those of domestic graduates. A telling practical point, however, is that the FMGs have not made those choices of location and specialization that might have established them as indispensable to the social goals toward which corrective legislation came to be addressed.

The Health Professions Educational Act of 1976, passed on 10 January 1977, is rapidly changing the pattern of FMGs' entry into the United States. Congress passed the act because it considered there was no longer an insufficiency of physicians in the United States, and that there was no further need for preferential immigration arrangements for alien physicians. Further, it intended that future emphasis should be on the production of primary-health-care physicians and on the improvement of services to health-manpower-shortage areas.

Underlying the policies directed at the FMGs were two other concerns: first, that the quality of the educational preparation of many FMGs was lower than should be accepted in the United States; and second, that migration to the United States drew important resources from the developing countries. This legislation addresses the quality issue by specifying much more stringent qualifying examinations: the ECFMG is replaced by the Visa Qualifying Examination (VQE), which is the equivalent of parts I and II of the U.S. National Board Examinations; an English proficiency examination is also required. The quantity issue is dealt with in several ways: by limiting access to exchange-visitor status by requiring the examinations mentioned above, and by limiting the period of its validity; and by a change in the preferential status of physicians under the general immigration regulations.

What will be the effect of this legislation? First, the total number of FMGs coming to the United States for training will be sharply reduced. Prior to this legislation, the figure was about 7,500 per year; a 66 percent decrease, bringing the figure to about 2,500 per year, is projected. About half of these will have passed the VQE and language-proficiency tests. The remainder will enter under family-preference immigration regulations.[7]

Given that FMGs coming to the United States for postgraduate training will decrease by 5,000, what will be the impact on U.S. institutions? Expanding domestic medical education will only partly meet the shortfall. By 1981, there will be an estimated 20,000 first-year medical-residency positions in the United States, and a domestic graduating class of 16,800. Assuming alien FMGs will bring the number of filled residencies to about 19,000, a gap of 1,000 positions will remain.[8] These vacancies will not be evenly distributed, of course, but will be concentrated in certain localities and types of hospitals. This gap is recognized as an important public-policy problem. The hospitals that have depended on the flow of FMGs for house staff will find these changes difficult to adapt to, and even disruptive.

The Department of Health, Education, and Welfare has been exploring ways of handling the impact of the legislation. To begin with, a waiver was obtained to defer until 31 December 1980 the application of the regulation requiring prior arrangement of affiliation with a training institution and the examination for language proficiency. Meanwhile, affected institutions are being given a schedule for phasing down their requirements for FMGs, and are being encouraged to take steps that will reduce their dependency on FMGs. Such steps might include: improving residency programs so as to attract more U.S. domestic graduates and USFMGs; shifting emphasis from inpatient to ambulatory care, so as to reduce the need for physicians; and increasing the use of physician extenders such as nurse practitioners and physician's assistants.[9]

Waivers and phase-downs notwithstanding, the clear intent of this new policy is to eliminate the exchange-visitor route as a significant source of interns and residents for U.S. institutions and, more generally, to reduce U.S. reliance on alien FMGs as a source of physician manpower.

USFMGs—The Migrant Physicians of the 1980s

One aspect of the FMG problem that is not discussed by the authors of this book, and that does not appear to be addressed by those responsible for implementing the legislation, has to do with USFMGs. This is already a problem for the families involved: Young people rejected from medical-school entry in the United States yearn to become physicians by any means; they accept the risk of going abroad for a medical education of uncertain quality; and they then search for professional reentry into the United States, particularly for good clinical experience and, ultimately, for residency training and licensure.

The forces internal to the United States that have attracted foreign physicians over the past two decades remain, despite the legislation. In particular, the effective economic demand for physicians will remain well in excess of the supply. Here we see another manifestation of the manpower market at work: Large numbers of medical-student candidates willing to pay substantial tuition fees for a medical education are a powerful force for generating medical-education programs. In response, increasing numbers of foreign institutions are developing medical-education programs to attract U.S. citizens, the most recent being in the Caribbean.

Looking ahead, the principle enunciated by the authors might well apply: Any nation that restricts its production of physicians while its effective economic demand for physicians is well in excess of supply risks the possibility of attracting FMGs, or of having its own citizens go abroad for training and then return. The stage would seem to be set for at least the latter event in the United States. While immigration regulations may close the door on FMGs, no such door is available for closing on the USFMGs. Qualifying examinations and licensure procedures are the available measures of control, but those seem unlikely to be major barriers to reentry.

It is possible that the flow of physicians to the United States through these channels could rival the earlier flow of FMGs from the developing countries. It is at least a matter for serious attention.

Conclusions

One of the more interesting aspects of physician migration has to do with the international context in which it occurs. Indeed, the more important insights into the problem are derived from that international framework.

For example, the push factors at work in the LDCs find their full meaning only in relation to the pull factors in the MDCs; each set of forces finds its strength only in relation to the other.

The same is true of the concept of effective economic demand for physicians. While there are domestic effects of a low or high EED, the effects on international physician migration must, of course, be felt in an international market. The United Kingdom, for example, is both a recipient of migrant physicians, particularly from Commonwealth countries, and a donor to Canada and the United States. The United Kingdom's EED lies between those of countries that send it their physicians and those that receive them from the United Kingdom. Thus, the United Kingdom's problem as both a donor and a recipient can be understood only in this international arena.

It is important that lessons taken from such international relationships influence public-policy decisions. In the LDCs, a narrowly placed domestic view of the problem of physician shortages worsened by emigration might well stimulate a decision to increase investments in medical education as a means of repairing the shortage. Lessons from the international setting would instruct policy makers that such investments could be wasteful, and might actually serve to accelerate outward migration.

On the U.S. side, the legislation restricting the entry of FMGs is expected effectively to close the door on traffic of physicians from medical schools abroad. Observations drawn from the international context, however, suggest that the forces that drew so many thousands of FMGs to the United States have not been changed in a major way by the legislation. Only the point of entry has been affected. The pulling forces are still there, and the possibility exists that the United States' own students, who are immune to the immigration restrictions of the recent legislation, may respond by flowing in substantial numbers to foreign medical schools and returning as USFMGs. Here again, public policy made domestically should not be blind to lessons that can be drawn from the international arena.

Notes

1. *Rural Development.* Sector Policy Paper. (Washington, D.C.: World Bank, 1975), p. 19.

2. Ruth Leger Sivard, *World Military and Social Expenditures 1977* (New York: Rockefeller Foundation, 1978).

3. John H. Bryant, *Health and the Developing World* (Ithaca, N.Y.: Cornell University Press, 1970), p. 49.

4. Ibid., p. 267.

5. Ibid., p. 177.

6. *The Role of Foreign Medical Graduates in U.S. Graduate Medical Education Programs, 1976 and 1977* (Chicago, Center for Health Services Research and Development, American Medical Association, 1978; mimeographed).

7. Internal documents, Department of Health, Education, and Welfare, January 1978.

8. Ibid.

9. Internal documents, Department of Health, Education, and Welfare, January 1978.

Appendix Immigration and Licensure Policies in the United States

Throughout this book, there have been illustrations of the manner in which the progressive liberalization of immigration policy in the United States has influenced the inflow of FMGs to the nation's health-care system. The following discussion is an attempt to shed more light on: (1) the nature of the changes in immigration policy, and how they have affected physician migration; (2) the role of the Exchange Visitor Program as a part of immigration policy; (3) the relationship between immigration policy and corresponding developments with respect to medical licensure in the United States; and (4) current legislation pertaining to health-manpower development in the United States.

Early Immigration Policies

Before 1819 there was practically no restriction on the flow into the United States of people from other countries. In that year, however, the government enacted a law requiring the captain of each vessel entering a port of the United States to provide port authorities with an account of the vessel's passengers.

From 1820 until the end of the century, the inflow from northern Europe predominated, augmented in turn by that from central and southern Europe and, during the middle years of the nineteenth century, by an inflow of people of Asian origin. In 1880 Congress, desirous of putting an end to immigration from the Orient, passed the first of several "Chinese Exclusion Acts" and made a "gentleman's agreement" with Japan that attempted to bar the entry of Japanese to the United States.

While such laws effected a considerable decline in immigration just prior to and during World War I, the new waves of immigrants beginning to arrive thereafter led to the passage, in 1921, of America's first Quota Act, to which was added, in 1924, a visa system which, in theory as well as in practice, gave preference to immigrants from the Western Hemisphere, particularly those from northern Europe. While immigration did not decline immediately after 1924 (there were nearly 200,000 immigrants each year until 1930), the characteristics of the immigrants changed somewhat. During the years of the economic depression, however, conditions both in the United States and elsewhere were not propitious for migration, and thus the inflow to the United States declined until after World War II, when it started to increase again at a rapid rate. [36]

Immigration Policies and Foreign Students

In 1936 the government of the United States, in an effort to promote better understanding among nations, launched a program involving the mutual exchange of students. As part of this policy the United States signed the Convention of Buenos Aires, which contained articles encouraging the exchange of students between the United States and the countries of Central and South America. [36] This was followed by the Fulbright Act of 1946, which reemphasized the government's policy of promoting international goodwill and understanding through students. This act authorized the Secretary of State to establish a program of international exchange by: (1) financing studies, research, library operation, and other educational activities of (or for) American citizens in schools and institutions of higher education in foreign countries; (2) financing similar activities for citizens of foreign countries who were enrolled in American schools and institutions of higher learning located outside the United States and its territories (for example, the American University in Beirut), including payment for transportation, tuition, maintenance, and other expenses related to scholastic activity; and (3) furnishing transportation for citizens of foreign countries who wished to attend American schools and institutions of higher education located in the United States. This program was funded by the revenue from the State Department's sale of surplus goods and supplies left in foreign countries after World War II. This revenue took the form of a credit in the foreign country, and could not be converted into U.S. currency. [49]

Implementation of the Fulbright Act not only turned out to be a powerful instrument of American foreign policy, but also relieved somewhat the mounting pressure on American universities to accomodate the thousands of war veterans whose education had been either interrupted or postponed by the war, and to whom the government had granted an entitlement to higher education, either in the United States or elsewhere. This legislation was of particular interest and concern to the American medical profession which, under the aegis of quality, was disinclined to view favorably any measure that might result in the expansion of enrollment in medical schools, the shortening of the duration of medical education, or changes in the curriculum.

The international program for educational and cultural exchange was broadened in 1948 by the Smith-Mundt Act, which authorized the appropriation of federal funds, to be used jointly with available foreign currencies, for the development of a real two-way exchangc. To facilitate the entry of foreign students to American universities, the Smith-Mundt Act authorized a special category of visa, the Exchange Visa or J visa. The act stipulated that students could enter the United States as nonimmigrant visitors, and would be allowed to stay until the termination of their studies. Because of the limited number of places for students in undergraduate medical-education programs in the United States, the Exchange Visitor program did little to accommodate foreign students who wanted to obtain basic medical education in the United States. It is noteworthy that, to this day, relatively few foreign students have received basic medical education in the United States, compared with the many Americans who have qualified abroad. On the other hand, given the burgeoning internship and residency programs in the United States, the Exchange Visitor program soon became a vehicle for expanding graduate medical education and, at the same time, for meeting the growing need for staff in hospitals—although neither of these was the intended purpose of the Exchange Visitor program as it applied to medical students.

It is worth noting at this point that the rapid expansion of hospital internship and residency programs was partly due to the large numbers of American World War II veterans seeking specialty training before returning to practice. It was also due, in part, to the relatively large number of new hospitals, and the expansion of facilities in many others, that resulted from the Hill-Burton Act of 1946, which authorized federal support for hospital construction. By 1950, however, the number of veterans seeking graduate training had declined. In addition, because of the Korean War, many young American physicians who might otherwise have been undergoing graduate training were on active military duty. Thus many hospitals were left with unfilled positions that they were reluctant to abolish. [49] The role of the FMG in making up that deficiency is now a matter of history. Moreover, with the knowledge that they could have manpower that was less expensive than fully trained physicians, many hospitals had further expanded their graduate training programs and had organized campaigns for the deliberate recruitment of physicians trained abroad.

Initially, the Smith-Mundt Act placed no time limit on a foreign student's stay in the United States. Thus, during the early years of the Exchange Visitor program, little notice was taken of the fact that many were staying much longer than the time their education was generally expected to require, and that some of these were becoming permanent residents. To counter this, the Smith-Mundt Act was amended in 1956; those with J visas were thereby required to leave the United States for at least two years before being eligible to apply for either an immigrant visa, a nonimmigrant visa, or an adjustment of status to that of permanent resident. To all intents and purposes, this regulation turned out to be just another of the various regulations governing the Exchange Visitor program that had to be circumvented; the number of waivers requested and granted to foreign physicians mounted rapidly. Moreover, many who were unable to obtain waivers did not return to their homelands (as intended by the law) but went instead to other countries, particularly Canada, where they could readily find employment until such time as they could legally reenter the United States. For those doing so, the country concerned thus became a "way station" for immigration to the United States.

The two-year restriction related to reentry of foreign physicians became a focus of controversy in the 1960s, in view of the divergence of two distinct policies with respect to foreigners that existed in the United States at the time. On the one hand was the policy to promote the international exchange of education, for humane as well as political and economic purposes; the idea was that students would return to their homelands, both to serve there and also to counter what the U.S. government considered unwarranted propaganda unfavorable to the United States. On the other hand was the recognition that the United States needed many more physicians than the medical-education system was producing. The ramifications of the controversy surrounding FMGs' length of stay in the United States are spelled out in a study sponsored by the U.S. Department of Health, Education, and Welfare. [49] In short, the issue centered on the State Department's proposal that the Immigration and Nationality Act be amended to allow foreign physicians to enter the United States on the grounds of alleviating the country's manpower problems, rather than on the pretext of education. It is noteworthy that both the AMA and the AHA opposed this proposal. The AMA contended that the temporary admission of foreign physicians for the purpose of filling the service needs of hospitals through internship and residency positions would adversely affect the standards of both medical education and the care of hospitalized patients. The AMA advocated, instead, a time limit on the stay of FMGs in the United States, and enforcement of the provision that they leave the country for two years before reentering. The AHA, on the other hand, contended that the United States should increase domestic production and, to this end, suggested federal funding for the construction of additional medical schools and the renovation of existing ones, as well as federal grants for medical education—policies that the AMA had been opposing all along.

The outcome of the debate was, in essence, that from 1970 onward everyone possessing a J visa had the right to apply for a change to immigrant status, and that it was no longer necessary to leave the United States during the period of the changeover. Many foreign physicians almost immediately took advantage of that ruling, as is evident from statistics presented earlier in this book.

Changing Policies toward Immigration

The Exchange Visitor program was one of two predominant visa programs running in parallel, the other one enabling foreigners to be admitted directly as immigrants. Until 1965 this program was administered according to the Quota Act of 1921, which largely favored countries of the Western Hemisphere, particularly northern Europe. This act was replaced by the Immigration Act of 1952, which somewhat broadened the quota system as originally conceived.

In 1965 the immigration law was again changed, and with the change the national-origins-quota system was abolished. Accordingly, as from 1968 onward, immigrants were to be admitted on the basis of the order in which they applied for visas, regardless of country of birth. Additionally, total annual immigration was not to exceed 290,000, including no more than 120,000 annually from the Western Hemisphere (the remaining 170,000 from other parts of the world) and no more than 20,000 annually per foreing state. An annual quota of 17,000 was established for professional and highly skilled personnel in preference categories 3 and 6 (those having an exceptional ability and those who represented skills that were in short supply in the United States). Foreign physicians potentially fell into one or the other of these two categories.

One result of the 1965 amendment to the immigration law was not only a rapid increase in the total number of foreign physicians entering the United States as immigrants, but also a rapid change in the characteristics of the immigrants in terms of nationality. This is shown in the following figures, which reflect the changing percentage distribution of physicians and surgeons admitted to the United States as immigrants, by country or region of last permanent residence. [49]

	Percentage for Fiscal Year		
Country or Region	*1957*	*1965*	*1971*
Asia	7.8	10.2	66.6
Canada	12.9	18.9	8.2
Cuba	10.0	10.0	1.7
Mexico	4.8	5.5	0.5
South America	11.5	17.3	4.7
United Kingdom	7.1	7.3	4.7
Europe, excluding United Kingdom	36.6	20.9	8.0
Other	9.3	9.9	5.6
Total	100.0	100.0	100.0
N	1,990	2,012	5,756

It is not clear why some foreign physicians initially entered the United States as immigrants, while others came initially as exchange visitors (primarily as students in graduate training programs). In both cases, the individuals concerned have had the option of returning to their country, or at least of leaving the United States. Moreover, since 1970 exchange visitors have had the option of converting to immigrant status without first having to leave the United States for two years in order to do so. To a large extent, this provision negated a ruling by the Immigration and Naturalization Service that foreign interns and residents were restricted to the J visa. In any case, there appear to be marked differences in the mode of entry used by physicians from different countries. For example, in 1971 physicians from Latin American countries seemed highly disposed to enter as exchange visitors, while those from Asian countries (except Japan) were more inclined to enter as immigrants. [49]

Between 1962 and 1970, on the average, about 24 percent more physicians entered annually as exchange visitors than as immigrants. Beginning in 1971, however, the proportion entering as immigrants began to rise and even to surpass the proportion entering as exchange visitors. As explained previously, part of this rise resulted from the conversion to immigrant status on the part of an increasing number of foreign physicians who had initially entered the United States as exchange visitors; that is, many physicians were taking advantage of the 1970 ruling in this regard. All other intents and purposes notwithstanding, the ways in which the 1965 law concerning immigration, and the 1970 law concerning exchange visitors, were administered effectively encouraged the direct immigration of foreign physicians, and assisted graduate medical students of foreign nationality to remain in the United States upon completion of their training.

Licensure Regulations

While the government's concern was to liberalize immigration policy in order to help the nation meet its need for skilled manpower, particularly physicians, professional associations of American medicine were concerned about the quality of medicine and were also afraid that the market for physician services would become more competitive as greater numbers of foreign physicians entered that market, particularly if they entered as fully licensed physicians. Thus, as immigration policies became less restrictive, policies concerning full licensure became progressively more restrictive. At the same time, there appeared to be a tendency to allow more physicians to practice with less-than-full licensure. The discussion that follows is largely based on a study of state licensure policies that was supported by the U.S. Department of Health, Education, and Welfare. [12, 15]

As early as 1938, the AMA's House of Delegates had passed a resolution declaring that United States citizenship should be required of all FMGs. Many state licensing boards adopted this requirement. In addition, or alternatively, a number of state boards required either an immigrant visa or a declaration of intent to become a citizen. During the period 1953–1975, the states frequently altered their requirements for full licensure, the tendency being generally toward a relaxation of requirements that had little to do with competency. By 1975 only five states (Montana, New Hampshire, South Carolina, Wisconsin, and Wyoming) continued to require that FMG applicants for full licensure either be, or submit a declaration of intent to become, citizens of the United States.

During the same period, the number of states requiring FMGs seeking full licensure to pass a special basic-science examination also decreased significantly, from seventeen in 1953 to seven in 1975, with six of the latter prepared to waive the requirement under certain circumstances (Colorado being the exception).

A growing number of states have made postgraduate training a prerequisite for full licensure, and have stipulated that this training be pursued in programs approved by the AMA. The primary mechanism for screening foreign applicants for these programs has been the examination administered by the ECFMG. Since its introduction in 1957, thousands of FMGs have taken that examination, which has been administered both in the United States and in a number of other countries throughout the world. While the examination has made full licensure more accessible to qualified FMGs throughout the United States, it has also helped to increase the number of FMGs in the United States who are without a full license but are practicing medicine with what may be called less-than-full licensure. Among these are many who have tried and failed the examination, and are thus known to the AMA, and others (perhaps as many or more) who entered the United States before taking the examination and have still not taken it. These would most probably be unknown to the AMA, and thus form part of the medical "underground."

Nine types of less-than-full license are currently available in the United States. Of these, the five under which FMGs are likely to practice are those that authorize practice: (1) in educational settings (postgraduate training programs); (2) in government institutions under state, county, or municipal control; (3) in medically underserved areas as designated by state boards; (4) in faculty positions in medical schools; and (5) in any situation, including private practice, until naturalized citizenship is attained, at which time full licensure is conferred.

In 1953, only two types of less-than-full license were available to FMGs, namely, the educational and governmental licenses, and these in only twelve states. During the next twenty years, the underserved-area, faculty, and citizenship-related licenses appeared for the first time, while the number of states authorizing educational and governmental licenses doubled.

The license allowing practice in postgraduate training programs was the most widely used less-than-full license throughout this period. The greatly increased use of this license appeared to be related to the increased specialization of physicians, requiring longer periods of postgraduate training. Given that a greater number of physicians who were practicing in lengthy training programs were either not yet eligible for full licensure or had planned to practice in a state only for the duration of their training, state boards recognized the need to provide legal status for these trainees through the use of less-than-full licensure for educational purposes.

During the period under review there was a significant increase in the use of less-than-full licenses in government institutions, which, being generally less attractive to USMGs, have come to rely heavily on FMGs.

The use of the less-than-full licenses for practice in shortage areas began in 1959, with only one state using it in any given year during the period 1959–1969. By 1975, six states were using it.

The requirements and time limits pertaining to less-than-full licensure vary from state to state, and from one type of practice to another. Those in the educational area usually include only ECFMG certification and permit practice only until the completion of postgraduate training. Those in government institutions vary from one extreme to the other, including, in a few cases, full licensure, and in a few virtually no specific requirements. It has been suggested that the variety of the requirements for employment in government institutions indicates that states may be using the less-than-full licensure rather flexibly, as a means of alleviating manpower shortages in less attractive areas of work.

Current Policies on Health-Manpower Development

On 12 October 1976, the government of the United States signed into law the Health Professions Educational Assistance Act, which aims essentially at producing more primary-care practitioners and improving health services in manpower-shortage areas. [56] The law, which was effective as of 10 January 1977 and will remain in force for at least five years, declares that there is no longer an insufficient number of physicians and surgeons in the United States, and that there is no further need to accord preference to alien physicians and surgeons with regard to admission to the United States. More specifically, the act indicates the following:

1. Foreign physicians wishing to enter the United States as immigrants on the basis of their professional skills (preference categories 3 or 6 of the

Immigration and Nationality Act), as special immigrants from the Western Hemisphere, or as nonpreference immigrants must pass parts I and II of the National Board of Medical Examiners' examination (or an equivalent) and be competent in written and oral English.

2. A foreign physician may enter the United States as an exchange visitor (J visa) only on condition that:
   a. a school of medicine and an affiliated hospital have agreed in writing to provide his training;
   b. the individual, in addition to meeting the previously mentioned requirements, will be able to adapt to the educational and cultural environment in the United States and will have had adequate prior training;
   c. the individual has a commitment to return to his country and his country has given, in writing, an assurance that on completion of training he will be appointed to a position where his acquired skills will be utilized fully;
   d. the individual will stay in the United States no more than two years, unless additional training is specifically requested by his country.

   (The requirements pertaining to exchange visitors may be waived until 31 December 1980, in situations where there might be a substantial disruption in the health services provided by the graduate training program in which the alien seeks to participate. However, in granting waivers, the Attorney General must ensure that the total number of aliens participating in such programs any time after 10 January 1977 does not exceed the number participating on 10 January 1977.)
3. Foreign physicians who are in the United States as exchange visitors and who wish to apply for permanent-residence status are no longer eligible, simply on the basis of permission from their country, for a waiver of the requirement that they first return to their country for a period of two years.
4. Foreign physicians are no longer allowed to enter the United States as persons of "distinguished merit and ability" coming to perform services of an exceptional nature requiring such ability (H visa), unless they have a specific invitation, from either a public or a private nonprofit educational or research entity, to teach or to conduct research or both.

The act also stipulates important conditions under which substantial capitation grants will be made available to medical schools. For example:

1. Enrollments must not be reduced below the level existing in either the 1975–1976 or the 1976–1977 school year (whichever is the greater).
2. Schools must not reduce their levels of expenditure from nonfederal funds.

3. Schools must progressively increase residencies in primary care (family practice, general internal medicine, and general pediatrics) up to the level of 50 percent of residencies by 1980, and this must not be done at the cost of disaffiliating other residency programs.
4. Schools must reserve an "equitable number" of third-year class positions for the transfer of American citizens who were enrolled in foreign medical schools before 12 October 1976, who have completed two years of medical education, and who have passed part I of the National Board examination. The requirement for taking transfers may be waived if compliance would cause a school to lose accreditation or prevent a school from providing a high level of clinical training for added students because of an insufficient population served by the facility in which the school conducts clinical training. A school is not required to enroll any student who does not meet its entrance requirements (other than those related to academic or residence qualifications).
5. Residency training programs in family practice, general internal medicine, general pediatrics, or general obstetrics and gynecology, in order to receive federal assistance, must establish a "reasonable number" of positions that can be shared by an average of two trainees per year. Among other things, this would make it possible for women trainees with children to complete residency programs on a part-time basis.

The act also authorizes, among other things:

1. Grants to individual schools of medicine for the purpose of establishing and maintaining an academic administrative unit to provide clinical instruction in family medicine. The unit must be comparable to those of other major clinical specialties in terms of status, faculty, and curriculum. It must control a three-year residency program in family practice, with the capacity to enroll a total of at least twelve interns or residents a year.
2. The broadening of grants for training in family medicine (previously limited to hospitals) to include schools of medicine or osteopathy, or other public or private nonprofit entities. Authority is added to train physicians to teach family medicine, with traineeships and fellowships to be awarded for such physicians.
3. Grants and contracts to schools of medicine to plan, develop, and operate approved medical-residency programs in internal medicine or pediatrics that emphasize training for practice in general internal medicine or general pediatrics. Traineeships and fellowships are authorized for residents participating in these programs.
4. Contracts with schools of medicine to plan, develop, and implement Area Health Education Center (AHEC) programs. At least two other

health-science disciplines must participate, and at least 10 percent of the respective school's undergraduate clinical education must be conducted in an AHEC or at locations under its sponsorship. At least one AHEC in any AHEC program must provide for or conduct a medical-residency training program in family medicine or general internal medicine, with no fewer than six individuals in first-year positions. A physician's assistant or nurse practitioner program must be included.

5. Grants or contracts to schools of medicine to meet the costs of planning, developing, and operating or maintaining programs for the training of physician's assistants to deliver health care, with the training to last at least one school year, to consist of supervised clinical practice and at least four months of classroom instruction, and to have a minimum enrollment of eight students per program.
6. Grants and contracts to medical schools to assist students from disadvantaged backgrounds to enter and complete medical education.

The act authorizes the expenditure of about $2,700 million, during a four-year period covering the fiscal years 1977 through 1980 inclusive, for the development of health manpower to serve the nation's needs, with the focus on underserved populations. The award of National Health Service Corps scholarships and loans by the government will be contingent on the awardee's willingness to serve for a minimum of two years in a manpower-shortage area. At the request of the awardee, service may be deferred for up to three years of internship, residency, or other advanced clinical training. The penalty for failure to perform obligated service will be three times the amount of scholarship assistance, plus interest at the maximum rate prevailing, to be payable in one year. No relief is to be available under bankruptcy law until five years after payment has become due.

Students of medicine will be allowed to borrow up to $10,000 a year, and a total of $50,000, to be used solely for tuition and other reasonable educational expenses, including fees, books, and laboratory equipment. No more than 50 percent of students in each class of a medical school can be borrowers under this program. Borrowers may enter into agreement with the Department of Health, Education, and Welfare for the repayment of loans, plus interest, at a rate of no more than $10,000 a year for each year of service in the National Health Service Corps. or in private practice in a manpower-shortage area.

The act has evoked a variety of reactions in the United States. The AHA, for example, concerned about a potential severe reduction in services at some big-city hospitals, has asked: (1) that the implementation of the act be delayed until 1978; (2) that the government establish an advisory panel to develop criteria for waivers regarding foreign physicians entering the United States as exchange visitors; and (3) that FMGs be allowed to take the

ECFMG examination as a temporary equivalent to the National Board of Medical Examiners test.

Medical-school authorities are reported as protesting the probability that federal funds will be withheld from institutions that fail to accept, as transfer students, Americans who have been studying abroad. At stake in the confrontation are tens of millions of dollars in funds and guaranteed student loans, which the law says will be forfeited by medical schools that do not agree to go along with this and other parts of the plan for the improvement of health services in manpower-shortage areas. Hitherto, most of the federal funds granted to medical schools were for research and the training of research workers. The new law focuses instead on the use of funds for the training of larger numbers of manpower for the delivery of primary care.

Various reactions to the act have also been manifested among the large colony of foreign physicians in the United States, many of whom have acquired membership in the American College of International Physicians, Inc., an association of foreign physicians founded in the United States in 1975 with the aim of helping its members attain and maintain acceptable standards of proficiency and satisfactory working conditions.

Reactions have also been evident among physicians in other parts of the world, many of whom, taking advantage of the ninety-day period between the promulgation of the act and its implementation, hastened to enter the United States during that period. It is said, for example, that an estimated 220 South African physicians availed themselves of this opportunity. [9] It is also reported that between 300 and 400 physicians working in the United Kingdom's National Health Service hurried to meet the deadline of 10 January 1977. Many of them, once they have established residence and registered in the United States, are expected to return to the United Kingdom to complete their commitment to the National Health Service, and then emigrate to the United States within 364 days after their initial departure from the United States. A number of those involved are physicians who came to the United Kingdom from India and Pakistan. [26]

References

1. American Medical Association. Medical education. *Journal of the American Medical Association* 210 (1969): 1455–1582.

2. American Medical Association, 76th Annual Report. Medical Education in the United States 1975–1976. Appendix 1. *Journal of the American Medical Association* 236 (1976): 3049–3055.

3. American Medical Association. Center for Health Services Research and Development. *Foreign medical graduates in the United States, 1970,* edited by J.N. Haug and B.C. Martin. Chicago: American Medical Association, 1971.

4. American Medical Association. Center for Health Services Research and Development. *Profile of medical practice; reference data,* compiled and edited by S.G. Vahovich and P. Aherne. Chicago: American Medical Association, 1973.

5. American Medical Association. Center for Health Services Research and Development. *Profile of medical practice, 1974.* Chicago: American Medical Association, 1974.

6. American Medical Association. Center for Health Services Research and Development. *Profile of medical practice, 75–76,* edited by J.R. Cantwell. Chicago: American Medical Association, 1976.

7. American Medical Association. Center for Health Services Research and Development. *Socioeconomic issues of health, 75–76,* edited by H.R. Mason. Chicago: American Medical Association, 1976.

8. American Medical Association. Division of Medical Education. *Directory of approved internships and residencies.* Chicago: American Medical Association, various years.

9. Ashford, N. 'Exodus' of whites worries South Africans. *The Times* (London), 8 January 1977.

10. Association of American Medical Colleges. *Graduates of foreign medical schools in the United States. A challenge to medical education.* Washington, D.C.: Association of American Medical Colleges, 1974.

11. Attah, E. Medical school development in Nigeria. *Journal of the American Medical Association* 234 (1975): 1275–1276.

12. Butter, I. *Foreign medical graduates: a comparative study of state licensure policies.* NCHSR Publication no. (HRA) 77-3166. Rockville, Md.: U.S. Department of Health, Education, and Welfare, 1977.

13. Butter, I. The migratory flow of doctors to and from the United States, *Medical Care* 9 (1971): 17–31.

14. Butter, I., and Schaffner, R. Geographic mobility of foreign medical graduates and the doctor shortage: A longitudinal analysis. *Inquiry* 9 (1972): 25–33.

15. Butter, I., and Sweet, R.G. Licensure of foreign medical graduates: an historical perspective. *Milbank Memorial Fund Quarterly* 55 (1977): 315–340.

16. Bowers, J.Z., and Rosenheim, Lord, eds. *International conference on the migration of medical manpower.* New York: Josiah Macy, Jr. Foundation, 1971. Papers from an International Macy Conference.

17. Bryant, J. *Health and the developing world.* Ithaca, N.Y.: Cornell University Press, 1969.

18. Conferéncia Pan-Americana de Educacao Médica (VI) y Congresso Brasileiro de Educacao Médica (XIV), Rio de Janeiro, 1976. Masificacion estudantil. Paper prepared for the conference by Juan Carlos Casiraghi.

19. De Vise, P. Physician migration from inland to coastal states: Antipoda examples of Illinois and California. *Journal of Medical Education* 48 (1973): 141–151.

20. Dublin, D. Foreign physicians: their impact on U.S. health care. *Science* 185 (1974): 407–414.

21. Educational Commission for Foreign Medical Graduates. *Annual report, 1974.* Philadelphia, Educational Commission for Foreign Medical Graduates, 1976.

22. Fein, R. *The doctor shortage: an economic analysis.* Washington, D.C.: Brookings Institution, 1967.

23. Flexner, A. *Medical education in the United States and Canada.* Report to the Carnegie Foundation for the Advancement of Teaching. Bulletin no. 4. New York: Carnegie Foundation, 1910.

24. Goldblatt, A. et al. Licensure, competence, and manpower distribution; a follow-up study of foreign medical graduates. *New England Journal of Medicine* 292 (1975): 137–141.

25. Haug, J.N. and Stevens, R. Foreign medical graduates in the United States in 1963 and 1971: a cohort study. *Inquiry* 10 (1973): 26–32.

26. Hebert, H. Doctors rush to beat US residence deadline. *The Guardian,* 21 December 1976.

27. Henderson, G. *The emigration of highly skilled manpower from the developing countries.* New York: United Nations Institute for Training and Research, 1970.

28. International Bank for Reconstruction and Development. *Health: sector policy paper.* Washington, D.C.: International Bank for Reconstruction and Development, 1973.

29. International Bank for Reconstruction and Development. *World Bank atlas.* Washington, D.C.: International Bank for Reconstruction and Development, 1973.

30. International Labour Office. Tripartite World Conference on

Employment, Income Distribution and Social Progress and the International Division of Labour. *Employment, growth and basic needs: A one-world problem.* Report of the Director-General of the International Labour Office. Geneva: International Labour Office, 1976.

31. Kleinman, J.C.; Brandt, U.C.; and Weiss, R.J. Postgraduate training and work experience of non-ECFMG certified physicians in the U.S. *Medical Care* 13 (1975): 205–208.

32. Kleinman, J.C.; Weiss, R.J.; and Felsenthal, D.S. Immigrant physicians. Results of a cohort study. *Inquiry* 12 (1975): 193–203.

33. Kleinman, J.C.; Weiss R.J.; and Felsenthal, D.S. Physician manpower data: the case of the missing foreign medical graduate. *Medical Care* 12 (1974): 906–917.

34. Lowin, A. *FMGs? An evaluation of policy-related research.* Prepared for the National Science Foundation, Washington, D.C. NSF-C814. Minneapolis: Inter Study, 1975.

35. Luft, H. *Determinants of the flow of physicians to the United States.* Santa Monica, Calif.: Rand Corporation, 1970.

36. Margulies, H., and Bloch, L.S. *Foreign medical graduates in the United States.* Cambridge, Mass.: Harvard University Press, 1969.

37. Medalie, J.H. The present and future of primary medical care in Israel. *International Journal of Health Services* 2 (1972): 285–295.

38. National Science Foundation. *Scientists, engineers and physicians from abroad; trends through fiscal year 1970.* Surveys of Science Resources Series, NSF 72-312. Washington, D.C.: National Science Foundation, 1972.

39. Oteiza, E. Emigración de profesionales, técnicos y obreros calificados Argentinos a los Estados Unidos—análisis de las fluctuaciones de la emigración bruta, Julio 1950 a Junio 1970. *Desarollo Economico* 10 (1970–1971): 429–454.

40. Pan American Health Organization. Study Group on Health Research. *Health research in Latin America.* Scientific publication no. 275. Washington, D.C.: Pan American Health Organization, Pan American Sanitary Bureau, Regional Office of the World Health Organization, 1973.

41. Paredes-Manrique, R., and Agualimpia, C. *Study of human resources for health and medical education in Colombia: methods and results.* Bogota: Ministry of Public Health and Colombian Association of Medical Faculties, 1972.

42. Rodriguez, M.I. El estudiante de medecina—su distribución en las Américas, 1971–1972. *Educación Medica y Salud* 8 (1974): 360–389.

43. Ronaghy, H.A.; Zeighami, E.; Farahmand, N.; and Zeighami, B. Causes of physician migration: responses of Iranian physicians in the United States. *Journal of Medical Education* 51 (1976): 305–311.

44. Senewiratne, B. Emigration of doctors: a problem for the developing and the developed countries. II. *British Medical Journal* 1 (1975): 669–671.

45. Stevens, R. *American medicine and the public interest.* New Haven, Conn., and London; Yale University Press, 1971.

46. Stevens, R.A.; Goodman, L.W.; and Mick, S.S. The "Medical Underground." Some thoughts and a reply. *Medical Care* 13 (1974): 440–443.

47. Stevens, R.A.; Goodman, L.W.; and Mick, S.S. What happens to foreign-trained doctors who come to the United States. *Inquiry* 11 (1974): 112–124.

48. Stevens, R. et al. Physician migration reexamined. *Science* 190 (1975): 439–442.

49. Stevens, R., and Vermeulen, J. *Foreign trained physicians and American medicine.* DHEW Publication no. (NIH) 73-325. Bethesda, Md.: U.S. Department of Health, Education, and Welfare, 1972.

50. Stevens, R., and Vermeulen, J. *Foreign trained physicians and American medicine.* DHEW Publication no. (NIH) 73-325. Bethesda, Md.: U.S. Department of Health, Education, and Welfare, 1972.

51. Symposium on the Foreign Medical Graduate in the United States Health Care System, 14–17 January 1975. *Report.* Palo Alto, Calif.: Sun Valley Forum on National Health, 1975.

52. United Nations Conference on Trade and Development. *The reverse transfer of technology: its dimensions, economic effects, and policy implications.* Geneva: UNCTAD, 1975.

53. United Nations Educational, Scientific and Cultural Organization. *Foreign students in medical schools.* Statistical study prepared by the UNESCO Office of Statistics in collaboration with Huguette Leiler. Paris: UNESCO, 1974.

54. United States. Bureau of Health Resources Development. Office of International Health Manpower Studies. *Foreign medical graduates and physician manpower in the United States.* DHEW Publication no. (HRA) 74-30. Bethesda, Md.: U.S. Department of Health, Education, and Welfare, 1974.

55. United States. Department of Commerce. Bureau of the Census. *Statistical abstract of the United States, 1975. National data book and guide to sources.* Washington, D.C.: U.S. Department of Commerce, 1976.

56. United States. Department of Health, Education, and Welfare. Health Resources Administration. Bureau of Health Manpower. *Fact sheet: Health Professions Educational Act of 1976* (*PL94–484*). Bethesda, Md.: U.S. Department of Health, Education, and Welfare, 1976.

57. United States Department of Health, Education, and Welfare. Public Health Service. Health Resources Administration. Bureau of Health Resources Development. *The supply of health manpower: 1970 profiles and projections to 1990,* DHEW Publication no. HRA 75-38. Washington, D.C.: U.S. Department of Health, Education, and Welfare, 1974.

58. United States. Department of Health, Education, and Welfare. *Health manpower source book.* Public Health Service Publication no. 263, section 9. Washington, D.C.: U.S. Government Printing Office, 1959.

59. United States Department of Health, Education, and Welfare. Public Health Service. Health Resources Administration. National Center for Health Statistics. *Health resources statistics reported from the National Center for Health Statistics 1975.* Rockville, Md.: U.S. Department of Health, Education, and Welfare, 1976.

60. United States. Department of Health, Education, and Welfare. Public Health Service. Health Resources Administration. Bureau of Health Planning and Resources Development. *Trends affecting U.S. health care system.* DHEW Publication no. (HRA) 76.14503. Rockville, Md.: U.S. Department of Health, Education, and Welfare, 1976.

61. United States. Library of Congress. Foreign Affairs Division. Congressional Research Service. *Brain drain: a study of the persistent issue of international mobility.* Prepared for the Subcommittee of National Security Policy and Scientific Developments of the Committee on Foreign Affairs, U.S. House of Representatives. Science, Technology, and American Diplomacy series. Washington, D.C.: U.S. Government Printing Office, 1974.

62. Weiss, R.J. The effect of importing physicians—return to a pre-Flexnerian standard. *New England Journal of Medicine* 290 (1974): 1453–1458.

63. Weiss, R.J. et al. Foreign medical graduates and the medical underground. *New England Journal of Medicine* 290 (1974): 1408–1413.

64. Williams, K.N., and Brook, R.H. Foreign medical graduates and their impact on the quality of medical care in the United States. *Milbank Memorial Fund Quarterly* 53 (1975):549–579.

65. Williams, K.N., and Lockett, B.A. Migration of foreign physicians to the United States: the perspective of health manpower planning. *International Journal of Health Services* 4 (1974): 213–243.

66. *World almanac and book of facts 1977.* New York and Cleveland: Newspaper Enterprise Association, 1976.

67. World Health Organization. *Equivalence of medical qualifications and the practice of medicine: a survey of existing legislation.* Geneva: World Health Organization, 1967.

68. World Health Organization. *Multinational study of the international migration of physicians and nurses: statistical enquiry.* Unpublished information.

69. World Health Organization. *World directory of medical schools 1970.* Geneva: World Health Organization, 1973.

70. World Health Organization. *World health statistics annual 1972,* vol. 3. Geneva: World Health Organization, 1976.

71. World Health Organization. *World health statistics report,* no. 27, 1974. Geneva: World Health Organization, 1974.

72. Yankauer, A., and Arias, J. *Studies of the migration of Colombian medical graduates. I. Secular trends and permancy of migration to the USA.* Unpublished document.

Index

About the Authors

Alfonso Mejia is a graduate of the National University Medical School, Bogota, Colombia, and received the M.P.H. from The University of Pittsburgh. He has served in various capacities in the Colombian Ministry of Health, and as head of the Department of Community Medicine, National University, Bogota. He is currently chief medical officer, Health Manpower Systems, Division of Health Manpower Development, World Health Organization. He has published many articles on health administration, epidemiology, and health-manpower problems.

Helena Pizurki received the B.Sc. in education from the University of Maryland and has taught in public and private schools in the United States and Switzerland. Formerly a full-time staff member of the World Health Organization, she is now a consultant to its Division of Health Manpower Development.

Erica Royston received the B.Sc. in economics from the London School of Economics and has worked as an economist and statistician in England and Switzerland. Ms. Royston is currently a statistician in the Division of Family Health of the World Health Organization.